MW01137862

The Thigh Gap Hack

By

Camille Hugh

PUBLISHED BY:

FeminineContour Publishing

Copyright 2013

" When I cracked open your book and began reading it I started to cry. They were tears of joy because for a woman who has been bottom heavy my entire life I felt for the first time I was reading something that was real and true.

Since implementing some of the diet and exercise tips in your book I can notice my thighs getting smaller and I can finally see and feel between my legs. Now that's sexy.

Before reading your book I was apprehensive to follow it because it goes against everything doctors, nutritionists, and fitness professionals recommend. I myself am an AFAA certified group exercise instructor, and sat there scratching my head wondering why I'm not getting it right and why I could not sculpt the body I desire and help other women do the same.

So I've tried that and its help me lose 2% body fat and 22lbs in a month. Not that I'm big on numbers or anything because I dread getting on the scale. I feel good being able to cross my legs comfortably and having a visible waistline. And yes I think it's sexy to be able to start to see my thighs gap.

I also stopped doing heavy weights on my lower body, and the forward lunges that were bulking me up. I'm only 25 years young; I don't want to be anorexic by any long shot. What I want to be is healthy so that I can increase my lifespan and hopefully impart some good into the world before my time is up.

What I like about you is you are smart, and you have done your research. You are not afraid to go against the opposition. You're not selling women a bunch of BS that leaves them more frustrated than before they started."

- Brandy, North Carolina (Real Customer)

"This is a book geared toward women who want to look healthy and have slim thighs in the process. It speaks of healthy eating and exercising. I bought the book because I work out a lot and wanted to know of exercises that can strengthen my legs without giving me bulky, over developed muscles. Given the fact that clothes are geared toward women who are very tall and have very thin skinny legs, it's no wonder women want to work on this particular body part."

- Maria L (Real Customer)

"'The Thigh Gap Hack' reveals many workouts that you may not have otherwise known to trim down your thighs as opposed to squats and leg lifts which, ultimately, just make them bigger. It it a user-friendly instruction manual to achieving the thigh gap every girl wants without starving themselves to death!"

- Erin B (Real Customer)

"I find great motivation in your work and your amazing progress. Every time I feel like giving up, I know that it´s going to be worth it if I keep strong. It´s because you know what it´s like to be so close to achieving your goals, but struggle with your own body for months, and because, even though it is incredibly hard, you can actually make it! "

- Samantha, New York (Real Customer)

BOOKS BY CAMILLE HUGH

The Thigh Gap Hack Diet - *Includes 30 Recipes*

Lose Water Weight and Look Great in 15 Days or Less (June 2014)

WORKOUT   VIDEOS   BY   CAMILLE   HUGH

Bye-Bye Thunder Thighs (March 2014)

The Thigh Gap Hack Workout (June 2014)

Pop Cardio Dance Videos (youtube.com/thighgaphack)

To receive updates, advanced notice and special deals on the release of the above projects, sign up at http://www.thighgaphack.com/vip

http://www.thighgaphack.com

License Notes

This book is licensed for your personal enjoyment only. This book may not be re-sold or given away to other people. If you would like to share this book with another person, please purchase an additional copy for each recipient. If you're reading this book and did not purchase it, or it was not purchased for your use only, then please purchase your own copy. Your support and respect for the property of this author is appreciated.

http://www.thighgaphack.com

YOUR FREE GIFT

I'd like to reward you with FREE access to my premium Fitness Newsletter.

You'll learn my best cutting edge strategies for getting lean and lowering your body fat on a busy schedule, how to reprogram your genetics, and get "insider" tricks picked up from the world's elite fitness trainers. Get free instant access to the excuse proof fitness survival guide and newsletter today.

To sign up visit www.thefemininecontour.com or www.thighgaphack.com/freegift

Disclaimer:

Copyright 2013, All Rights Reserved

No part of this publication may be reproduced, transmitted, transcribed, stored in a retrieval system, or translated into any language, in any form, by any means, without the written permission of the author. Understand that the information contained in this book is an opinion, and should be used for personal entertainment purposes only. You are responsible for your own behavior, and this book is not to be considered medical, legal, or personal advice. Nor is this book to be understood as putting forth any cure for any type of acute or chronic health problems or psychological illness. The programs and information expressed within this book are not medical advice, but rather represent the author's opinions and are solely for informational and education purposes. The author is not responsible in any manner whatsoever for any injury or health condition that may occur through following the programs and opinions expressed herein. Dietary information is presented for informational purposes only and may not be appropriate for all individuals. Consult with your physician before starting any rigorous exercise program or altering your diet.

TABLE OF CONTENTS

WHAT THIS BOOK IS FOR

This book is meant to give you in depth researched and tested, advanced techniques that will help you lose stubborn body fat and/or muscles in the area of the inner and outer thighs.

THIS BOOK IS NOT FOR

Those looking for validation to develop an eating disorder, those with an eating disorder or unhealthy relationships with body image and food.

PART I – The Thigh Gap Defined

THE FEMININE BODY

Have you ever heard of the "Golden Ratio"? It is, in mathematical terms, a comparison of any two aspects that leads us to proportion them in the ideal way. Algebraically, if you have two numbers, A and B, it has to be such that (A + B) divided by A = A divided by B.

Mostly, the golden ratio has only been associated with facial beauty. Basically, the idea is that the human face has ideal measurements and ratios in relation to each other that make someone beautiful. Generally, the more proportionate the features on the face, the more attractive the individual is said to be. While everyone is special in his or her own way, beauty, in the eyes of many beholders, appears to be reducible to a definitive formula. Logically, we can explain why Brad Pitt or Halle Berry are considered universally beautiful, and others are universally seen as not.

If there can be such a thing as an ideal face, that the overwhelming majority of people find attractive, surely there is such a thing as an ideal body. Well, as it turns out, there is. The supposed ideal ratio is between 0.69-0.72, dividing the waist measurement by the hip measurement where the waist is 69% to 72% of the hips (e.g., a 70cm waist and 100cm hip). Others have said .7 and less, but it is suffice to say as you move away from the ideal, fewer and fewer people will find your body pleasing.

Our brains are programmed to look for symmetry and balance everywhere. We are attracted to it and try to create it in design, beauty, nature, animals, cosmology, mathematics, and the list goes on. This means that what we consider a good body is really based on what we view as a body that projects certain characteristics and bodily symmetry.

When it comes to the "ideal" shape for women, femininity (think curves) and proportionate measurements reign. Slender shoulders, wider bust, narrow waist that cinch in, hips no wider than the bust, and lean legs that taper in. Unfortunately, many of us have bodies that defy us as we try to get this ideal shape.

Think about pear shaped women, where the hips and thighs are much larger than the upper portion of the body, apple shaped women, where the tummy and waist are much larger than the lower body, and banana shaped women, where there are no curves to speak of, denoting a lack of femininity.

Getting the body to optimum proportions is no easy and straightforward task, particularly when it comes to leaning out the lower body as opposed to the middle because of a complicated host of reasons, but it can be accomplished. I can say this with confidence because I have completely reshaped my own wider hips and thighs, as well as those of countless clients, through my online body contouring and nutrition program, The Feminine Contour. (www.thefemininecontour.com)

In doing so, I've face palmed many a time upon clients spouting the craziest myths and bad advice as truth. As a result of the cloud of confusion surrounding contouring the ideal, feminine, proportionate figure, many women have sadly resigned themselves to believe in the false conclusion that the body they truly want will always be out of grasp.

Can you imagine how frustrating that is to someone who knows from experience that not to be the case? While I can reach my female friends, family and clients, the fact is more people need and want this information than I can reach face to face, and it would be a disservice to keep it under wraps. Furthermore, it would be much easier to recommend this book, rather than continuing to dole out the same advice over and over, several times per week.

So when I am asked, "Why write another diet/fitness book?" my response is, "This isn't another diet and fitness book!" Other books on the market have simply ignored what women have been shouting at the top of their lungs for eons, and that is the need for a clear and finite solution to reducing inches from the inner and outer thigh to reveal a slender (not muscular, bulky, strong-looking or thick) thigh and leg. Oh, and the quicker the results, the better, of course!

Now, I'm well aware the mere mention of purposefully not trying to build muscles lifting heavy things or doing 15 minutes of high intensity training as a complete workout is not en vogue at the moment and thus automatically makes this book controversial. However, in my opinion, the pendulum has completely swung in the fitness world to trainers trying to convince women they should want something they do not want or to use methods that won't get them where they want to be.

When my journey to change my body began, my goal was to research and find the answers to the questions that the fitness trainers wouldn't even acknowledge, much less answer, so that I could finally stop spinning my wheels. I'm proud to be able to take all I've learned and share it with women like you, who may be currently stuck in a fitness rut and desperately seeking direction.

If you've been working towards a "perfect body" as defined by most women and men, and having some success from taking wild stabs in the dark, think about what this means for you. This book of resources and tools means that now you can select your workouts, follow a diet based on your specific desires, and get the results you want. There is no longer a need for time consuming and demoralizing trial and error where you may take one step forward and two steps back simply because you don't know any better.

You won't have to hop on every bandwagon that comes around because you'll have a simple blueprint laid out right before you within these very pages. You'll be able to share your newfound knowledge with other women and prevent them from the frustrations you know only too well. Best of all, you'll finally know what it feels like to be happy and confident in your skin because you will look the way you want to look. Finally, should you ever deviate you'll be capable of getting back to perfect (if your idea of perfect is in alignment with what I've been referencing so far).

WHAT IS THE THIGH GAP?

A thigh gap is precisely what it sounds like, a gap between the thighs. The caveat is that gap must be visible when standing completely upright with the feet placed firmly together. Oftentimes, the bevvy of pictures of people on the Internet displaying their gaps are not true thigh gaps, but optical illusions. In other words, what you may be seeing in pictures are women and girls standing with their legs and feet apart or sticking out their buttocks and slightly bending forward with turned out heels in order to create the appearance of a gap.

However, that's only a camera trick, and a good one at that if you instantly want to appear to have slimmer hips and thighs in photographs. What we are going after in this book is a more permanent solution. Why settle for only looking good in photographs when you can feel and look awesome in real life, right?

I only mention the imposters because the critics are quick to paint wannabes as a testament to the thigh gap being an unrealistic goal. They cry that the images are not real, and that the models are airbrushed and sticking out their backsides to trick you into thinking this goal is achievable. I've even read of one Doctor who claimed only pre-pubescent girls were able to have the gap and that it was a signal of malnourishment. Yet, these insensitive and loud proclamations are hardly proof that there aren't plenty of women and girls walking around with real gaps who are not malnourished, pre-pubescent or anorexic. Additionally, from even the very last row at any fashion show, anyone can see that plenty of models really are as slender in real life as they appear in print and on television.

I left out an important factor in defining the thigh gap above, and since you are not blinded by extremism, you've probably noticed that all thigh gaps are not created equal. They can range anywhere from a small to wide space in between the thighs, or even just a keyhole at the top of the thighs. Even the tiniest of gaps qualifies you and can make all the difference in how feminine and sexy your legs appear and you feel.

One last point I'd like to address is an argument you will often hear opponents of the thigh gap state the first chance they get. It's the idea that you don't have to be skinny or slim to have a thigh gap, as there are overweight and fat women with gaps due to their wider hips.

Indeed, even a broken clock is right twice a day. I wholeheartedly agree that having a gap won't put you in an exclusive club of skinny-only women and thus shouldn't be the standard of which thinness/skinniness is measured. However, the part where critics try to connect not defining your fitness level by your gap to discouraging women from trying to get one because fat women can have them too, leaves me befuddled.

My clients and most women are not trying to look like the overweight women with natural thigh gaps. Furthermore, women willing to work out and diet to achieve a thigh gap are looking for the trim figure sure to accompany the application of those methods. The ones who are already fit are doing it because they prefer the way it looks. Like it or not, fatter thighs usually means stretch marks, dimples, cellulite and jiggly, loose skin have a greater likelihood of being present. Most women desire the slim and firm inner and outer thigh that can be found on slender women with thigh gaps. I suggest you ignore the red herring and treat this diversion tactic for what it is, a non-factor.

You may think I'm preaching to the choir here, but in the instance critics decide to read this, I thought I'd take the opportunity to clarify a few things. Hopefully the above will also serve to enable you to engage anyone in debate should you choose to do so, but moreover, reassure you that you're not liable to give credence to people's opinions when it comes to your body.

What follows is my arsenal of rules that I have developed, discovered and perfected over the years. Experimentation, reading and deciphering tons of scientific studies and having an insatiable appetite for learning every trick that can be applied towards body contouring has been quite literally my obsession. I like to call these methods hacks due to their lesser known status, departure from the conventional and ability to generate results in the fastest way possible, but you still have to put in the work nonetheless, as with anything in life, to see results. Adapt and follow these tricks and you will be well on your way to contouring the svelte, model-like body that you've been dreaming of.

CAN ANYONE GET A THIGH GAP?

Unequivocally, the answer to this often asked question is a resounding yes! According to some "experts", a thigh gap is unattainable unless you have wide set hips, which are genetically predetermined and cannot be altered. Therefore, they say it is worthless to try and achieve the goal of sleek, thin thighs unless you are born with the bone structure. Of course they conveniently omit any indication of how one would know if her body were indeed properly structured, since it is difficult to tell when carrying an excess load of body fat.

I would advise not giving any merit in the statements of those who have never succeeded, much less attempted, to do what you want to do. The impossible is limited to what we have seen and I have seen what these experts say is impossible. The fact is, trying to get a thigh gap is highly frowned upon and discouraged as it is unfairly linked with women and girls who idolize and want a thigh gap so badly that they are willing to go to extreme lengths, such as chronic exercise coupled with starvation or some other form of eating disorder to achieve it.

Of course, there is more than one way to skin a cat, and just as some people take unhealthy and extreme approaches to reach their weight loss goals, there are equally a large number of individuals who opt for the healthy and safer techniques. Keep in mind, that there are also so many varying degrees of thigh gaps and a plethora of different aesthetic looks when it comes to the 'gap' that one could be trying to achieve, that asserting such a blanket statement is frankly, laughable.

The truth is, technically, any woman can get a thigh gap if they lower their body fat and get skinny enough. Obviously, if you have narrow hips and strive for a smaller gap, your goal can be more easily attained than if you have narrow hips and strive for a larger space between your thighs. The way most women's bodies work is that when they lose weight they tend to see the results in their upper body (arms, face, back and abs) way before the weight starts to come from the lower body (hips, thighs, butt, legs). That is what is commonly referred to as 'stubborn body fat'.

It's called stubborn because the fat seems to want to cling on in these areas while easily melting away in other areas. The best analogy I've heard likened losing stubborn body fat to emptying a pool. Before you can touch the water in the deep end, you first have to get rid of the water in the shallow parts. You can thank Mother Nature and your hormones for this! Much to many women's chagrin, the female body wants to store fat for childbearing purposes – even if you have no intention of bearing children in the near future.

The trick to achieving a thigh gap, or just a slimmer, more proportionate lower body then, is to obliterate the stubborn body fat. Fat cells have two types of receptors: Alpha-receptors, which inhibits the breakdown of fat, and Beta-receptors, which stimulate the breakdown of fat. Unfortunately, women have more alpha-receptors in the hip and thigh region.

To add insult to injury, women also have three to five times more lipoprotein lipase, an enzyme that stimulates fat storage in their lower body than their upper body. Can you now see why these areas are typically the first place in which women gain weight and the last place they lose it? Hopefully you are starting to realize why the best defense is offense when it comes to accumulating fat in the lower body.

If you've been overweight all your life, you might think that the girls who have always been sensible about their diet and exercise have it easier, but think again. Even women already average to thin in their upper body will more than likely still need to lower body fat before the stubborn fat is targeted and affected. Trust me when I say that losing fat becomes harder the less fat you have to lose.

It's painfully clear the deck has certainly been stacked against us women, but before you go cursing the gods, just remember that the predisposition of women to store stubborn lower body fat is said to be for the protection of our reproductive organs, and it'll all come in handy one day as our bodies will be able to nourish itself during a pregnancy, if that is a goal. If not, let the cursing commence while you do what needs to be done anyway.

What else will determine how easy it will be for you to target and eradicate lower body fat or if you will like the majority who lose fat from everywhere else first and from their hips, thighs, and buttocks last? The answer is genetics. Genetics is your DNA that was inherited through genes passed on by one or both parents, and it mostly determines the pattern of weight loss.

In fact, scientists have discovered that the difference in fat distribution among women have a basis in the region and climate from which an individual's ancestors have come. For example, in hot countries, such as those within Africa or in the Mediterranean, women tend to store fat in the buttocks, hips and upper thighs, while individuals from certain Asian countries tend to store fat around the belly area.

It is thought that the body stores more fat in particular locations for those individuals who have ancestry in hotter climates because it would be more efficient this way than covering the entire body with layers of fat, which would affect the body's internal thermoregulation and make daily life unbearable.

For those individuals whose ancestry comes from cooler climates or Eastern European countries, the body fat distribution tends to be more even so as to insulate the entire body to bear the bitter winter months. I believe that cold thermogenesis also has something to do with why those who are exposed to cold store less fat and I will cover that in more detail soon. For now, I assure you that although genetics and hormones may not be on your side, you don't have to resign yourself to settling for an unsatisfactory body composition. It is completely possible to make a huge difference in your shape and tone your physique through exercise, diet, and a few well-placed hacks.

Once the stubborn fat goes, all that is left is the beautiful, toned muscle underneath. Without the excess fat on your inner and outer thighs, voila – your thigh gap will magically appear. And if it's any consolation, by the time you lose the stubborn fat on your inner and outer thighs and hips, the rest of your body will look absolutely amazing.

Having said all this, it would be irresponsible for me to advocate lowering your body fat into the dangerously unhealthy range, typically in the single digits for women, to achieve this look and therefore I obviously do not recommend that you do. That being said, I repeat, a major factor in whether or not you can get the aesthetic look of either an ever so slight part between your legs or a wider gap is based on the fat on the inner part of your thighs combined with your bone structure, so if you find your body fat getting too low for your taste through natural means, my chapter on outside hacks will be right up your alley. That's right, I've made sure 'The Thigh Gap' covers all the bases.

Naturally, you may be wondering just how lean or what weight you will need to be to reveal the results you want. Unfortunately, I cannot say because every woman is different. You may see excellent results once their body fat lowers to the 14% – 18% range. Meanwhile, some of you shorter and very petite girls/women may need to go a little lower before the gap makes an appearance. If you have wider set hips, it will not be necessary to get as lean as those with narrow hips because the gap will be apparent even with a little more fat padding due to your bone structure.

The main takeaway is fat is the common denominator and primary determinant of a thigh gap. Both narrow and wider hipped women can achieve this aesthetic with varying degrees of effort based on their goals. Should a woman with narrow set hips have the fat along the inner part of her thighs surgically removed via liposuction, it would result in the effect of a thigh gap, just as the narrow hipped woman who diets to get her body fat low enough that the fat from this part of the body melts off.

This is what is meant when I say that anyone can get a thigh gap. It may not be as wide as someone with the genetic predisposition, but if you shed enough of the fat, you will notice that your legs won't rub or touch when standing in a comfortable stance or walking, and there will be a space, albeit small if you have narrower hips, in between your legs. I say all of that to say, narrow hipped women, don't give up hope like the 'experts' advise you to!

The only reason you don't see more women leaning out this area of the body without struggling is not because women are incapable of doing so, but because interestingly enough, hardly anyone is offering the real solutions to the problem. I have no idea why this is, but I suppose it has something to do with the dearth of fitness experts being men and their training goals and problem areas being starkly different to women. I'd even venture to say most of the fitness 'experts' are unwaveringly focused on building up the body, and gaining more muscle as opposed to contouring it and dare I say, losing some muscle. In plain terms, they just don't understand.

Luckily, I do. I know all too well how frustrating it can be to have a legitimate problem and follow bad advice that only exacerbates it, or seek the answers only to find yourself being told that you should want "strong" legs and that "muscular thighs" are sexy. On top of that, it seems that any advice seeking for actually wanting to deliberately lose muscle is met with chastisement. Perhaps the incredulous idea that women have brains and are entitled to decide for ourselves how we want to look will squarely hit these trainers in the jaw when they start losing business for shabby results. I will gladly listen and take the business they clearly do not deserve.

Based on my clients and what I read on the message boards, I would purport that the majority of women don't want bulky, thick legs or find them sexy or appealing. Given the chance to slim out this trouble area, even if a wide gap is not achieved, they would be perfectly content. The good news is that I understand your frustrations and the physique you are trying to sculpt, so you can rest comfortably following my directions. Yes, I know for a fact that everyone is capable of thinning out their inner and outer thighs by following the techniques in this book.

IDENTIFYING YOUR UNIQUE PROBLEM

The first thing we need to do is figure out your unique problem so that we can address it appropriately. The two roadblocks to achieving the thigh gap are, as we've touched upon, fat (adipose tissue), and to a lesser degree muscle. Fat takes up a huge amount of mass, while muscles, especially if there is a large layer of fat over them, creates a thick, bulging look that is not conducive to the thigh gap.

Thus, to effectively slim down your thighs you are going to want to focus first on one thing, either losing fat, or losing muscle in the thigh region. There are different techniques one should follow depending on the immediate goal you are trying to achieve. Which applies to you? Let's find out now.

Whether or not you have hips that are wide set or narrow, you may have noticed that the inner, and possibly outer, part of your thigh is squishy to the touch and takes up a lot of mass. All too often, the first conclusion many women come to when they are unhappy with the size or all around mass of their thighs and legs, known as the circumference, is that they have too much muscle. Rarely is that the real cause of their unhappiness. This test will determine if the bulk of the mass on your thigh that is preventing you from having slender legs are due to fat or muscle.

First, extend your leg and stiffen or tighten your muscles. Pinch all around the area of your thigh including the upper, middle, sides, back and lower. If you are able to gather a lot of skin in between your fingers relatively easily, fat is the culprit. If you're still not sure, flick that area and if it jiggles loosely and moves around easily, again fat is your problem. If you are still not convinced, if you have a lot of stomach fat and cannot see the cuts in your abs, or if you fold your arms at the elbow at a ninety degree angle and your bat wings wiggle and jiggle, you don't need to focus so much on how to lose muscle but on how to target your body fat.

We've established your issue is having too many fat cells and adipose tissue, so I'm sure you want to know just how you should go about obliterating those fat cells. Diet is going to be a big part of your journey to a thigh gap, and I will have some great tips in the diet section of the book for you. The way you train will also be of major importance, especially if you have been training the wrong way or haven't been training at all because you've been trying to avoid building up more leg muscles, a common ideology and practice typically among beginners and novices.

Your main plan of action will be to reduce your overall body fat first through copious amounts of the right cardio and some resistance training, adopt a diet plan which will put you in a Calorie deficit (a Calorie is a unit of energy contained in our food that provides fuel for our muscles), and then, once the fat starts melting off revealing your muscles you can further stretch and tone the muscle underneath if you so desire.

I have to caution you against the prevalent mistake of endless leg-lifts and floor work where you focus on resistance training your legs because doing so will not be enough exertion of energy to get your heart rate up, which is non-negotiable when it comes to burning body fat. Doing this will only lead to the build up of muscles underneath the stubborn fat and that muscle will push the fat out further creating bulky, swollen looking legs.

The other thigh gap inhibitor for women, a major source of contention, is an over development of leg muscles. This is typically a problem in women who dabble in bodybuilding, have played sports that are taxing on the leg muscles, like soccer or gymnastics, or log a lot of hours in the gym using heavy weighs and resistance training with very little to no cardio. These women are already pretty fit by most people's standards with average to below average body fat, but despite their active lifestyle, find their hips and thighs proportionally out of sync with their upper body.

Muscular thighs are represented by an overdevelopment of (1) the hamstrings, which are the muscles at the back of the thighs that may have a prominent curve definition) and/or (2) the quadriceps, which are four large muscles at the front of the thigh.

These areas, especially when covered with fat, create a look that most women want to avoid due to its masculine like appearance as well as other negative byproducts, such as not being able to fit trendy styles of clothing with the prime example being the skinny jean. Particularly when it comes to jeans, while fatty thighs can be squeezed into the popular fabric, muscles are more compact and do not move as easily. Thus, women who are battling muscular legs find themselves having to purchase bigger jean sizes that may fit the thigh area and leave a lot of room in the waist or are baggy in the groin. Needless to say, this is not a good look.

If you want to be sure muscular thighs are your problem, tense your leg and try to pinch at the skin all around the thigh region, including the quads, back of the thighs and outer thighs. If you are not able to pinch or jiggle a lot of skin, then you can safely determine that muscular thighs is your issues. Also, if you tense your legs and a very defined curvature can be seen in your quadriceps and hamstrings, it is likely that you will want to focus on losing the muscles in your legs primarily, and put fat loss in the back seat.

To reduce muscular thighs and legs, you will have to drastically reduce the lower body resistance work and strain you may be used to putting your legs through when working out and opt to do other forms of exercise. It may be hard to resist the urge to cut back on training, especially when you get a high from feeling the burn in your legs, but you will have to do it to get your desired result.

If you are addicted to working out, like me, you may be wondering what you are supposed to do to really feel like you've gotten a proper workout? After all some of the bodies largest muscles are in the lower body and account for the biggest opportunity to burn calories. I will delve deeper in the upcoming chapters, but you don't have to worry about your workouts becoming so easy they become ineffective.

You will still be working out and maintaining your muscles, but in other areas of the body. Doing so will keep your metabolism humming along nicely. You will also still be incorporating lower bodywork in your workouts to burn extra Calories, however the moves will be more geared towards cardiovascular training and less hypertrophic. Finally, your main focus will be on your diet and what you consume after your workout to prevent anabolism (muscles getting bigger) and encourage catabolism (muscles getting smaller).

FINAL NOTE

Everyone has a different aesthetic and while there are some women who may scoff at the idea of trying to achieve a thigh gap, don't let their ideas of beauty discourage you from sculpting the body that will make you happy. Don't let them sway you with talk about how training and diet should solely be for strength and power purposes. You can diet and exercise with the sole intent to look good naked for yourself and your significant other!

One of the greatest deterrent to women succeeding in their diets is their fatter or skinnier female 'friends' ridden with Tall Poppy Syndrome and/or fat acceptance rhetoric. They are uncomfortable when you try to change because it's a constant reminder of their shortcomings or a threat to their perceived standing somehow. Remember that when they menacingly try to derail your diet or offer everything but support. Also beware of hypocrites who lash against the thigh gap, yet have no such negativity against those who want to lose muffin tops and bat wings or get six pack abs because they find those aesthetics appealing. The fact that you prefer the physical attributes you do is just as valid as long as you go about achieving that look without being destructive to your body, which is what I'm here to help you with.

I emphasize that there is nothing at all wrong with striving to look a different way than you do now, especially if you are currently at an unhealthy weight. The fat acceptance camp that encourages embracing your body, even if it's putting your life at great risk, permeates our society like a plague. If there are people around you who judge you or chastise you for wanting to look a certain way and you know that you are not harming yourself, you may want to reconsider whether or not they want the best for you and if you need those people in your life.

So far we have broken down what the thigh gap is, covered why anyone would want one, touched on the basic steps to achieve one depending on your unique problem and removed the roadblocks, which included discrediting the objectors, for you to begin your journey. Finally, the moment you have been waiting for - Let's get to the brass tacks of hacking the thigh gap.

PART 2 - Preparing For Success

GETTING STARTED

As with anything, in order to see whether or not progress has been made you need a reference point. Typically, the reference point is where you begin. I don't know about you, but the most fascinating and motivating part of someone's triumphant weight loss story is seeing before and after pictures. It's undeniable, tangible proof of how far someone has come and often a constant reminder to those individuals to never go back.

It is crucial that you take a before picture and weekly or monthly progress pictures of your body wearing the same clothing, as well as take measurements of your body so that you can see the subtle improvements to gauge whether or not you are on the right track. Another good reason to do this is so that you can send over your before and after pictures as proof to others that getting slimmer thighs and legs is accomplishable by following the hacks and techniques outlined in this book. Plus, once you have reached your goal of slimming down your stems, you should want to show off the fruits your labor has merited.

MEASURING YOUR THIGHS

You will need a measuring tape (preferably the flexible kind used for garments) and a roll of paper tape that won't pull your skin when removed. Paper tape is used for surgical purposes and if you don't already have some, can be found at your local pharmacy for a few dollars. The purpose of this is we want to clearly be able to see the gain that you make at the end of this process, or more precisely, see the losses!

You want to make sure to measure the same areas every time for an accurate picture of the transformation that will be occurring in your legs. The first part of the leg you will measure is directly above the knee. Wrap the tape around the knee without compressing the skin or drawing the tape too tight. There should be no bulging skin nor should the tape be too loose. Use a magic marker or pen and label the tape 'above the knee' for easy future reference.

The second part of the leg you should measure is the quadriceps. The best way to do this is to take a tape measure and hold it vertically along the length of the leg, starting from your pelvic bone to determine the exact locations of the thigh you will be measuring. I chose the pelvic bone because it isn't going anywhere and is easy to find by simply feeling around your hips, but you can also measure from the very top of the knee as well. If you choose to go with the pelvic bone as your base, feel for the groove or indentation in the bone and place the tape measure right into this groove.

Next, note with a marker the points on the thigh where you will take your measurements. You will want to take down the measurement for the upper inner thigh and the middle of the quadriceps. If you would like to be more precise, you can also take the measurement for the area right above the knee because you will see losses in this area following my protocol as well.

The final part of the leg that we want to measure is the area right at the beginning of the thigh, at the very top of the leg. Again, this is an obvious pocket where fat is stored and hard to get rid of. As you lower your entire body fat and conduct targeted exercises to firm up the area, you will be able to see the inches melt away.

These areas are the main spots we will be targeting to reduce the fat stores and/or muscle mass that have accumulated. When the pools of fat disappear you will have incredibly streamlined and feminine stems that you'll want to show off all day long.

Here's an example of what you should be doing. Start by holding the tape measure into the groove of the pelvis bone. You then determine you will subsequently be measuring the areas 6 inches (upper inner thigh), 10 inches (middle of the quadriceps), and 12 inches (area right above the knee) along the thigh. Make a dot on the thigh with a marker in all three areas and then proceed to measure those areas with paper tape or a flexible tape measure. Note the current measurements of the circumference of the thigh along with the corresponding lengths. Your notes should look something like this: 6 inches – 22 centimeters, 10 inches – 23 centimeters, 12 inches – 21 centimeters. Every time you update your measurements you will use those exact markers (6", 10" and 12" for example. Your numbers can and will vary depending upon your height and the length of your legs).

MEASURING YOUR BODY FAT

Again, we want to know what your body's starting point is so that we can measure the effectiveness of the program, therefore we want as accurate a reading of your beginning overall body fat as possible. The problem with most body fat tests is that your stats are being plugged into a formula based on a lot of assumptions about the standard composition of an average, American male or female. There is a lot of room for error when you are plugged into a formula, but you have to work around the errors by recognizing this fact and trying to get as close to the real numbers as possible. Below, I have provided multiple ways for you to have your body fat read.

HYDROSTATIC TEST

One of the most accurate ways to find out your lean mass and body fat percentage is to have a body composition test administered known as the hydrostatic test. With a margin of error of one percent, this test involves being submerged in water, not unlike a baptism. You are required to blow out as much air as possible, as any air can skew the numbers and increase your body fat percentage reading. The cost of such a test will set you back around $200. Many universities use this test primarily with athletes and will likely allow you to try it too, for a small fee.

SKIN FOLD TEST

The next test is the skin fold test. You are probably familiar with this test as it is readily available at almost all American High Schools and gyms. It involves pinching skin folds on different parts of the body such as the back, arms, love handles and measuring the folds that gather with calipers. The degree of accuracy for the results of a skin fold test varies due to the many different variables, such as the person administering the test, the quality of the calipers and how much skin is pinched.

The cost of the test is oftentimes free if you belong to a gym. Simply request that a personal trainer take your body fat reading and within 10 minutes or so you will have a result. If you are currently not a member of a gym, a little tip to get a free body fat reading is to stop into a gym and acquire one of the free guest passes that will give you access to the gym for a few days up to a week. This will usually afford you the opportunity to have a consultation with a personal trainer and you will have your body fat analyzed at no cost to you. If possible, try to get readings at 2 or 3 different gyms and take the average of the three readings.

BIOELECTRICAL IMPEDANCE TEST

Speaking of gyms, another test frequently offered there are bioelectrical impedance tests. For about $20 you will have an electrode attached to your hand and foot. After being still for a few seconds, the handheld device will send a painless signal through your body. The test works because lean body mass is mostly water and thus a good conductor of the current, while fat has little water and slows down the signal. The result will be less accurate due to factors such as hydration and food intake, resulting in a higher reading.

BOD POD

The Bod Pod uses air displacement to measure body composition. This test requires you not eat, drink or exercise two hours prior and involves sitting inside the closed egg in nothing but your underwear while the device measures your volume. The cost is anywhere from $30 to $40 and you can find locations that offer it by entering 'Bod Pod' for your city and state into any search engine.

INTEGRATIVE BODY COMPOSITION ASSESSMENT TOOL

The Integrative Body Composition tool costs $285 and includes a waist-measuring tape and caliper to measure the wrist. The concept of wrist measuring came from decades-old Swedish research that also looked at body makeup as a means to determine a healthy weight. Measuring wrists or knees helped researchers reach conclusions about whether someone had a larger or smaller frame.

Users get access to Health Profile Institute's software to add measurements such as height, weight, age and average exercise regimen for the past six months. This technique is said to be comparable in accuracy to hydrostatic weighing, more accurate than Bod Pod, and is more convenient and less invasive.

BATHROOM SCALES

There are bathroom scales where bioelectrical impedance analysis has been added that promise to give you readings of your body fat simply by sending a harmless electrical current up through your body to "read" the amount of fat body mass and lean body mass. These scales range from $50 to $100, but again hydration, or how much fluid in your body, can interfere with the accuracy of your reading. Little things like taking a shower before hand or your menstrual cycle can throw your number over by 5%, plus or minus! I would recommend you steer away or be very diligent about taking a reading right upon waking and before ingesting any food or drink.

DEXA SCAN

Finally, if your pocketbook is feeling a little heavy and you want the most accurate method available, you can turn to DEXA scanning. DEXA stands for "dual energy X-ray absorptiometry" and is the same imaging technology doctors will use to measure bone density. The test involves laying on an X-ray table for about ten minutes while a scanner measures your body fat, muscle and bone mineral density. Most major universities with solid exercise physiology research programs have these units, and will gladly provide evaluations to the public. Otherwise, some healthcare facilities have these units as they are used (and were originally developed) to measure bone mineral density. The cost ranges from $300 to $500.

TRACKING YOUR PROGRESS

Every week you are obligated to write down your progress until you reach your ultimate goal. Obviously, this means that you should have a goal in the first place. Some of you may say, well, my goal is to just have a thigh gap! I completely understand the logic, but it's always better to have concrete numbers, data and benchmarks along the way when trying to achieve a goal.

That's why runners keep track and have numerical goals for the times they run instead of just saying, "I want to run really, really fast". That is just too vague of a goal. How fast, in or under what amount of time, after how many weeks or months do you want to be able to do it in, how many days per week will you train to get to that point? That is the kind of detailed goal setting you should strive for.

Once your goal is in place, writing down your progress will do two things. First, it will hopefully keep you accountable and on track, so that you don't just stop doing the program. Most people are actually motivated by results, and at the smallest hint of success, which is only visible through tracking and documenting, hopefully you will be encouraged enough to stay the course and not give up as incremental change can be hard to spot with the naked eye.

Second, if you don't get the results at the end of this process you can go back, assess and examine if you truly followed the program and did what you were supposed to do. You can track where you made gains and where you experienced setbacks and then replicate the things you did to get progress and avoid those things that caused you to regress.

If you are unsure what your goal should be these tips will come in handy.

First, recognize that unrealistic and overly aggressive goals can undermine your efforts, so instead of striving to lose an unrealistic and dramatic lofty 10 pounds per week, keep the numbers confined to what is suggested as the healthy rate of losing weight, which is no more than 1 - 2 pounds per week. If you lose more, great, but if you lose weight too rapidly, this can lead to screwing up your metabolism which will lead to more problems down the road. We will cover the specifics of calorie intake a little bit later, but just keep in mind that your deficit should not exceed 1000 Calories per day.

You should also make your goal measurable. For example, specify how many miles and how long you are going to power walk each week to meet your calorie deficit goal, as well as which days of the week you will do which exercises and which days will be your rest days. Plan the times you are going to designate for working out down to the exact hour – from 5pm to 6pm or from 8am to 9am. Then, after you've finished your work out make note that you completed your task.

Explicit goal setting will also apply to your food consumption. In the chapter "Food Hacks", I will cover a very effective food hack that will require you to shift your Calories around per day, as well as some other techniques that will be very effective in facilitating a low body fat percentage. Not only will you need to set a goal of how many Calories you are to consume per week, you need to get down to the fine details and work out the numerical amounts per day.

The purpose behind all of the minutiae upfront is to remove the opportunity for you to make the wrong decision as you go. The more automatic you allow the process to become, and the less unsure you are of what you need to do, the better your chances are of sticking to your plan instead of deviating down the slippery slope of every day decision making. In fact, one productivity trick known amongst us life hackers is to remove as many opportunities to make decisions on the fly as possible.

If you have never heard of decision fatigue, this is the underlying reason why you want to set your goals in advance. The mechanics of decision fatigue states that the more decisions you make, the worst your decisions become. Thus, if you have to make a choice between good food choices, such as whole foods, vegetables, etc. and bad foods, such as sweet, carb filled products, all day – decision fatigue states that while your initial decisions will be to go for the good stuff, throughout the day and after being faced with more and more decisions, your choices will start to get poorer.

We do not want this phenomenon of devolving decision making to occur in this program, so we are going to remove the opportunities for you to make the wrong choices. If you know how many Calories you have to eat on Monday or if your meal is prepared and all you have to do is eat it, you will have a much easier time turning down those foods that will put you over your calorie limit.

Better yet, if you have a small list of all of your allowed foods/meal combinations, and studies have actually shown that we tend to eat the same foods over and over again with very little variety in between, the less chances for you to make a choice that will be counterproductive to your ultimate goal of thin and slim thighs.

Finally, I cannot stress enough, that in order to be successful and get the body you really want, you are going to have to ditch the diet mentality that relies on willpower and your ability to resist temptation. Instead, you are going to have to commit to permanent lifestyle changes. That means once you follow the procedures laid within these pages and are able to finally get the stubborn fat off your thighs and legs, you cannot go back to doing what you were doing before (or not doing) lest you revert to the way you looked before.

Behavioral changes can help put an end to the war against your willpower and allow eating and exercise to be healthful and enjoyable daily activities. Luckily, it takes approximately twenty-one days or three weeks of sustained activity to form a habit. But, if you never quite get there and you're still sneaking in the bad foods every week, or eating "replacement" foods, that will be your habit or way of eating forever. Additionally, if you never change your mind about the purpose of food and its relationship and effect to your health and appearance, you will go right back to your old eating habits sooner or later.

Some people manage to eat relatively clean, but think eating bad foods every now and then will be harmless. I don't want you to feel like you cannot enjoy good food, but those 'harmless' foods have been proven to cause addictive cravings for more of the same kinds of high fat, high sugar, high carb foods, which is what makes them anything but harmless.

Before you know it you'll be exercising a lot of willpower and potentially failing, as you face decision fatigue in trying to fight the urge to go back to your old comfort foods. Keeping these foods around or eating "replacement foods", like sugar-free ice cream, will cause your cravings for the real thing to stick around longer than had you buckled down and stayed away from the foods all together.

Once you have done all your initial measurements and embraced the mindset that results won't come magically and this desire you have for your body will take work, patience and diligence, you are finally ready to start. If you're reading this I know that you have probably tried all the conventional ways of slimming down your thighs only to yield the complete opposite results or none at all, and are set to do whatever it truly takes to get the svelte, feminine and proportional lower body you desire. I'm confident that you will put your all into this program and frankly, I can't wait to be bombarded by all of your success stories!

Part 3 – Popular Misconceptions

THE 80/20 RULE

Walk into any gym in America and you'll instantly realize there is no shortage of people furiously exercising in an effort to burn fat and lose weight. The stark division between men and women may make it difficult to tell depending on which area of the gym you frequent, but I would submit each gender makes up an equal number of gym subscriptions. When January 1st rolls around, good luck finding an empty treadmill, as losing weight is reported to be the number one New Year resolution[1]. Unfortunately, those same folks will probably still be at it the following year, and the next, because of their misguided beliefs about the role of exercise as a cure-all for fat loss.

---

[1] New Year's Resolution No. 1: Lose Weight, Doresett, Katherine, CNN www.cnn.com/2010/HEALTH/diet.fitness/12/31/lose.weight.new.resolutio n/index.html

In the exercise hacks portion of the book, I'll come back to the propensity for one half of the gym to have the majority of men lifting weights and the other half with the majority of women on the cardio machines and Pilates/Yoga mats, but our main concern at the moment is uncovering why exercise is not the holy grail for your fat loss.

Don't get me wrong, there is absolutely nothing wrong with exercise, but it is not the only or the most important component of sculpting your dream body. To obtain your desired physique, at the risk of being repetitive, we come back to FAT. If there is too much body fat, despite all of the Pilates, Yoga, weight lifting/toning exercises you may do, you will not get the svelte legs you want.

Please note I'm not giving you a free pass to abandon your workouts. According to the Mayo Clinic, exercise is a key element to maintaining weight loss and keeping your metabolism high[2], but you should know that while cardio and resistance training play a role in burning some fat and toning the body, your diet is the real star of the show.

In fact, a general rule of thumb is that losing fat is 80% - 90% diet and 20% to 10% exercise. Amazing, huh? It all makes sense once you understand that a non-negotiable element to weight loss is burning more calories than you consume. Since 3,500 calories equals about 1 pound (0.45 kilogram) of fat, you need to burn 3,500 calories more than you take in to lose 1 pound.

To put things into perspective, you would need to walk 64 minutes to burn off eating one doughnut, cycle 82 minutes to burn off the calories consumed by eating one Big Mac or jog 32 minutes for one order of Cheese fries. Granted, you shouldn't be eating those things if you want to get a thigh gap, but hopefully you can see how diet can sabotage your efforts for weight loss and body composition in spite of exercise.

---

[2] Mayo Clinic - www.mayoclinic.com/health/weight-loss/AN01619

For most people, it's almost impossible to eliminate the amount of calories through exercise that you could through dieting. Hence, it'd be easy to find individuals who have lost a lot of weight through diet alone, and much more difficult to find someone who has lost a significant amount of weight through exercise without controlling his or her diet.

I love how I feel after a good workout, but I would much rather eat cleaner than have to exercise myself to death, especially when exercising is only going to account for about 10% - 20% of my results. Also, there are so many tasty choices when it comes to clean food recipes to be found, one such source being my free newsletter, "The Recipe for a Thigh Gap" available at www.thighgaphack.com, that you don't even have to give up on one of the best things we have to enjoy in this life, good food.

If that isn't a compelling enough argument in favor of reigning in your diet instead of trying to out exercise poor food choices, another point to consider is the possibility to lose weight just from eating certain types of foods. You heard me right, it is possible to feed your body foods that can boost the function of your metabolism, as well as induce faster fat loss by eating your meals in a specific pattern such as calorie cycling, which we will delve into shortly. There are even foods you can eat which result in negative-calories, meaning you can eat as much as you want. Such eating strategies can drastically shed pounds that you won't be able to easily accomplish with exercise.

Finally, rounding out my case of why you should put more weight, pun intended, on your diet - too much exercise and exercise of the wrong kind can cause you to overly stimulate your muscles, which can leave you with the dreaded appearance of swollen, bigger thighs. Don't forget about the possibility of too much stress from exercise resulting in cortisol, a powerful hormone that is produced in the adrenal glands positioned on top of your kidneys, being released, which can lead to a perpetual catabolic state where muscle is broken down, and fat is stored.

I'm sure many would agree, there is nothing more frustrating than putting in the work in the gym only to see your problem area get worst. It can be discouraging and cause many women to give up hope.

In case I am losing or have lost some of you, I should preface this chapter by stating up front, I don't want you to think from now on you can only eat vegetables and drink lots of water. You already know doing those things will lead to fat loss; the problem is sticking to such a rigid diet gets boring and unbearable very fast. What I am about to reveal are honest and effective techniques and tricks that have been proven to rev up the metabolism and burn more fat, while still allowing you to eat heartily and not feel like you are going to die of hunger or starvation.

You won't have to force yourself to eat every few hours, nor get too crazy with counting Calories if you don't want to (I provide multiple options for you to choose from). Actually, what will likely happen is that you will find your hunger pangs and cravings finally begin to come under control. If you have struggled with a voracious appetite, you'll see it steadily decrease as you train your hunger.

If you're ready, let's dive into the hacker's way to eating for thinner thighs, lower body fat and ultimately a sleek and slim physique. I hope you're excited because as a budding hacker, you're about to learn how to do things smarter, not harder to get the same, if not better, results than going the conventional route.

FROM FOOD TO FAT

Fat gets a lot of flack, but the truth is we need some fat in our bodies. We are meant to eat and enjoy foods, as well as use food for nourishment. The problem arises when we pick "bad" foods and/or abuse foods either by overeating at individual meals or overall calories. I thought it'd be best then, to give you the skinny on fat and its relation to our hunger before going into how our first hack, Hunger Training™, can provide a remedy.

WHAT IS FAT?

Fat is an oily compound composed of the elements carbon, hydrogen, and oxygen. Carbon, hydrogen, and oxygen molecules bind together like links to form chains of fatty acids. When chains of fatty acids connect together with a molecule called glycerol, it's called a glyceride. Triglycerides, three fatty acid chains connected to a glycerol molecule, are the main type of fat in the foods we eat and in our bodies.

Our body fat serves many roles. It insulates us from the cold, pads and supports our vital organs, muscles, and bones, and is part of the structure of every cell membrane. It's an active organ, too. Fat cells behave very much like endocrine glands, secreting many different substances which are responsible for, among other functions, controlling and regulating appetite, blood pressure, some nervous system and hormonal signals, gene expression, and the formation of testosterone and some forms of estrogen. In short, fat cells are important organs with vital regulatory functions that help our bodies run smoothly.

The average person has around 35 billion fat cells stores in their bodies, but humans can have anywhere from 25 billion to 275 billion. Fat cells are microscopic, 10–20 times smaller than the diameter of a human hair (which is about 100 microns), but they are packed with energy. The average person has more than 100,000 Calories stored as fat on his body; that's theoretically enough fuel to jog close to 800 miles. Hopefully you can see why the claims of the body entering into starvation mode from eating 1200 Calories a day are pure rubbish. If you go hungry for a little while your body has a contingency plan.

Fat is stored in two primary ways - deep in the body cavities, and directly beneath the skin (called subcutaneous fat), and are kept in special compartments called adipocytes, a type of connective tissue often referred to as fat cells. Your genes determine where fat decides to settle on your body. You don't have any input or control over it. Women tend to accumulate it in the adipocytes on the hips, buttocks, and thighs, giving them more of a pear shape. This female pattern is also called gynoid, or gluteal-femoral pattern obesity. Men tend to accumulate it in the abdomen, giving them more of an apple shape.

WHERE DOES FAT COME FROM?

Forget about the widespread misconception of only dietary fat resulting in fat gain. Fat can come from all the foods we eat; that includes excess calories from protein, fat and carbohydrates. However, fat is the macronutrient that is most easily stored as body fat.

Every time you eat a food, bile and pancreatic enzymes in the small intestine digest it. The resulting fatty acids are then absorbed and transported to the liver where essential nutrients are removed. The rest is wrapped up and packaged together with proteins to form chylomicrons, so that it can travel through the bloodstream to all the organs and cells that need it.

The food will either get stored in the arteries of your heart, in your liver, or in the adipocytes on your hips, thighs, buttocks, or abdomen. Adipocytes love to store fat. They gobble it up like there's no tomorrow, and with the copious amounts many of us eat, most adipocytes in the United States are not lacking for fat.3

If you go on an eating spree, eating more food than your body needs in one sitting because your full signal doesn't kick in or you simply can't stop, a few things happen, none of them good. First, overeating increases the size of your fat cells and could cause you to gain more fat cells. Take my word when I say reversing fat cell enlargement is extremely difficult.

It should also be mentioned that overeating at any meal could cause an excessive surge in insulin, leading to more fat production, followed by a rapid drop in blood sugar, leading to

[3] Diabetes Self Management - www.diabetesselfmanagement.com/articles/exercise/burning_fat_thr ough_exercise/print/

cravings for sugar and carbohydrates. When attempting to lose body fat and weight, the one position you don't want to put yourself in is resisting these types of cravings.

Even more trouble occurs when your body decides to call upon its energy stores, because the body operates in real-time as opposed to a 24-hour period. There's this false idea among dieters that when the clock strikes twelve, the body calculates your deficit for the day and then burns that amount of fat. That's not quite how it works. Instead, your body takes what it needs from the food you give it and sets the rest aside for later as fat. You'll understand the dangers of overeating once you realize the body doesn't decide to only burn stored fat for energy.

Fuel for the human body takes three basic forms: carbohydrates (sugars), protein, and fat. Humans are capable of burning all three of these fuels, but do so at different times, rates, and under different circumstances. Almost all the carbohydrate eaten will be converted into glucose in the body. The only carbohydrates not changed to glucose are those that cannot be digested, like fiber.

In general, the body's pecking order for energy is glucose (carbs/sugars), then fats, and then proteins. Glucose is burned first because it is easier for our bodies to break down the molecules and digest them. Under the right circumstances (when carb stores are depleted and there is a calorie deficit or when you're exercising anaerobically) the body burns fat, as it is also a rich energy store. The body will burn protein as a last resort as it is not an efficient fuel source. Protein's main purpose is to build and repair tissue, not to provide fuel or energy.

To bring things full circle, when you eat more than your body needs in the moment, the excess gets stored as fat. As the body continues to be unnecessarily fed, it will not be encouraged to burn any of its stored fat for energy. Why should it bother digging out the fat stores for energy when it is being spoon-fed all day long?

Secondly, the spike in insulin, a storage hormone, from a large amount of food prevents fat burning from occurring and drives blood sugar down causing rebound hunger (you get hungry again soon after eating). You can surmise the more food you eat in one sitting, the longer the insulin sticks around. As if that wasn't enough, that insulin spike also interferes with leptin, the hormone secreted by fat cells that should tell the body to stop eating.

Finally, when your body does enter a metabolic state of using up energy, and this gets even more exaggerated when exercise is thrown into the mix, glycogen, fat, protein, muscle, etc. can be used as opposed to 100% of your fat stores. That means overfeeding could possibly result in some of excess calories that was stored as fat getting left behind.

Given all of the negative consequences listed for what can happen when you overfeed, it's easy to understand how you can put on weight when your hunger is broken and you wind up eating at a calorie surplus. However, there are probably some of you wondering what happens when you have a tendency to overeat at individual meals but still maintain a calorie deficit? While the consequences are not as bad, you still don't get off scotch free, because although you may wind up losing weight, not all of it will be fat.

LOSING WEIGHT VS LOSING FAT

Many people think 'losing weight' and 'losing fat' are interchangeable terms, but that is not the case. Losing weight means lowering your body weight, or the sum weight of your muscles, body fat, bones, organs, etc. Losing fat is lowering the amount of fat your body carries. Fat accounts for about 22% of the average male's body weight and 28% for the average woman, while an obese person has between 40% and 50% body fat.

Body fat levels common in the fitness industry is 10% body fat for men and 15% body fat for women, with many competitive body builders and trained athletes able to get their body fat down to 4-5% for men and 12 – 14% for women come competition time. However, these low competition levels of body fat and leanness are typically not sustainable year round.

To get a thigh gap, especially if you were not born with naturally wider hips or were dealt shorter limbs, fat loss and low body fat, more-so than weight loss, is paramount to your success. Even if you were born with wider hips but your thighs are too big for your liking, fat loss is going to be the key to getting your desired ideal trim looking lower body. Weight loss will undoubtedly come as you lose fat, but simply relying on weight loss alone is dicey. The reason being that your body weight is unreliable. It can fluctuate daily since it is influenced by water loss and retention, muscle loss and gain, your stomach/bowel/bladder contents and fat loss and gain.

Back in the day, the body mass index (BMI) used to be the standard doctors relied on when determining whether a body was a healthy size. BMI is a method that divides body weight in kilos by height squared, whilst taking no account of the person's fat to lean body mass ratio to determine whether their weight was to low, high or just right. That last line is one of the main problems with BMI.

Consider two individuals of the same weight and height who look entirely different from one another due to one having lower body fat. The person with the lower body fat will have a more toned and defined body composition. Needless to say this method is hardly used now. Instead, body composition, or the relative percentages of lean body mass and body fat in total body weight, is considered to be a more dependable source.

Going back to the consequences of overeating while still maintaining a deficit, your body adjusts to being deprived of food for a long period of time. It could turn to muscle for energy because it requires more to maintain than stored fat. The more lean mass (muscle) you lose, the lower your metabolic rate. The lower your metabolic rate, the lower your calorie deficit (food intake) needs to be to lose fat/weight.

Then when there is too large a surge of food at once, everything I previously mentioned for overeating on a calorie surplus happens: larger and increased fat cells, huge insulin spikes preventing fat burning until all insulin is cleared, higher propensity for fat storage, and 100% of fat not being burned when the body is in a metabolic state.

I say all of that to illustrate how you can lose weight and not lose fat when you're in a deficit but react to hunger by denying it for a major portion of the day and overeating at one or two meals. I make the bold assertion that if you are eating at a deficit for the day but overeat at meals, you need hunger training just as much as the person overeating at meals and eating at a calorie surplus.

Thus we can conclude from all we've learned that the most sensible way of eating is to (a) avoid overloading on energy (calorie intake) that is unable to be used by the body on a meal by meal basis to prevent calories being stored as fat in the first place, (b) make sure you use up all or most of the energy from your previous meal before eating again, and (c) eat in a matter that increases your metabolic rate to make sure you are burning up the calories that you put in your body.

PART 4 – Thigh Gap Hacks

HUNGER TRAINING™

I hope I've been able to make a compelling case for why you should no longer overeat at individual meals or in general. However, it's easier said than done when you're facing real or perceived hunger. That's where Hunger Training enters the picture. First, what is hunger? Hunger is not a singular motivation; it is the interaction of several different clinically measurable, provably distinct mental and physical processes.

Hunger training™ is a term I coined and developed into a program to tackle and conquer the difficult task of eating in moderation as well as learning how to eat for satiation (factors that make us stop eating) and satiety (factors that cause us to feel hungry or not hungry). There are those of us who have never had issues with knowing when to stop eating, while others of us have always been overeaters. Hunger training™ is for the later. If you sometimes eat despite not being truly hungry (e.g. - comfort yourself with food) or eat past the point of mindfulness because your full signals have been compromised, this hack is right up your alley.

Since following your current hunger signals stand to derail your fat loss progress, training your hunger will involve reorienting yourself with the feeling of true hunger and capping your individual meal calories in a tailored, calculated fashion.

Hunger training is such a rich topic that I can't fit everything about it in this chapter, which is why a full book on the subject is in the works (visit www.thefemininecontour.com/products to sign up for alerts on this upcoming project), but you will get the general idea behind the concept and tips to train your hunger as well as determine the amount of calories to consume per meal.

We've already determined that your diet is the integral link to losing fat. If your diet isn't in check, regardless of how much exercise you do, your dreams of a thigh gap will remain just that. On the flip side, your diet could consist of 100% "clean" whole foods; if you overeat on them, the scale won't budge in the direction you want it to. Therefore, you have to find a way to reset your hunger so that you are no longer hungry all the time and only seek nutritious food when your body needs it.

ALL ABOUT HUNGER

Hunger is a biochemical event that is controlled by an area of the brain called the hypothalamus. When a specific region of the hypothalamus is stimulated, hunger results. When a different area of the hypothalamus is stimulated, appetite suppression occurs.

Three hormones, insulin, leptin and grehlin, influence our hunger and satiety levels, and the macronutrients you eat, carbohydrate, protein and fat, strongly influence them. Ghrelin makes you feel hungry and leptin causes you to feel full. An easy way to distinguish between the two is ghrelin grows your appetite and leptin lowers it.

As blood leptin levels rise, and leptin increases in the brain, the hunger center of the brain deactivates, communicating you have adequate fuel, and diminishing the urgency to eat.4 On the other hand, when fewer leptin receptors are stimulated, the hypothalamus triggers our hunger and causes us to eat more food, which replaces our fat stores. Additionally, a drop in leptin can signal the body to slow the metabolism.

The scary part of having a broken hunger system, whether influenced by ghrelin or leptin, is hunger is a feeling that is hard to ignore, and it is quite difficult to distinguish between true biological hunger and everything else when food is just an arms length away.

Biological hunger is in your stomach and is expressed through hunger pangs or rumblings and grumblings. If you only ever received this signal of hunger, you'd be thin. The other "hunger" is mental or a phantom stomach that sends out signals of hunger in spite of your biological requirement for food. Some common triggers are when you are feeling emotional and stressed.

---

[4] Woodall, Robin Phipps. Weight-Loss Apocalypse: Emotional Eating Rehab Through the HCG Protocol

One way to tell the difference between the two types of hunger is phantom hunger comes on quickly, knows precisely what it wants (e.g. – cravings for a specific food), and wants a lot of it. Phantom hunger will drive you to go to almost any length to satisfy it. On the other hand, biological hunger comes on gradually and can be satisfied with relatively small amounts of food.

It is common for other protocols that involve reconfiguring your hunger to require you identify between when you are truly hungry and when you're dealing with phantom hunger. For example, you might be advised to wait out the phantom hunger until it gradually subsides, but I think this method has some shortcomings since people still tend to believe their phantom hunger is real when it doesn't subside as quickly as they'd like. Besides, this doesn't really help those who have the tendency to overeat to fill their biological hunger or eat regardless of realizing they actually aren't hungry.

The 'hack' in hunger training comes into play because you pre-determine in a proactive and precise manner when your body should be hungry (when you should need energy) and feed it just what it should need retroactively. Coupling this way of eating along with food choices that promote satiety, which increases compliance, will result in the body adjusting to its feeding schedule and phantom hunger making fewer appearances. Capping meal intake for a few months ensures some empirical confirmation of the appropriate amount of food for your needs and before you know it, you will be able to listen to your hunger cues naturally.

HUNGER TRAINING™ PROTOCOL

In order to begin Hunger Training™ you're going to need to invest in a really good heart rate monitor (HRM) (glorified pedometers and watchbands won't cut it) and a food scale. The heart rate monitor will be used to track the amount of calories you burn throughout the day and be the main indicator for how many calories shall be ingested at an individual meal (just enough calories your body needs), as well as the period of time between meals. The food scale will be used to determine the nutritional value of your meals.

Simply put, your individual meal calories will not exceed the amount of calories your HRM says you'll have burned and you will be required to wait until your HRM says you've burned off all of the previous calories supplied in the last feeding, before you will be permitted to eat again.

Be mindful that without the proper foods, which we will cover upon breaking down a few more hacks, your previous hunger pattern might indicate you are "hungry", but this scientific approach paired with filling foods will soon change that. If you're okay with the basic concept, let's go through each part of Hunger Training™, step by step.

The idea of hunger training came to me when I came across a study published in the British Journal of Nutrition, where a group of researchers found that the use of heart rate monitoring in the estimation of energy expenditure was a valid means of indirect whole-body calorimetry[5]. Once I learned the researchers used an ambulatory heart rate monitor that ~~provided minute-by-minute~~ heart rate throughout the day to

[5] Sana M. Ceesay, Andrew M. Prentice*, Kenneth C. Day, Peter R. Murgatryod, Gail R. Goldberg AND Wendy Scott, The Use of Heart Rate Monitoring in the Estimation of Energy Expenditure : A Validation Study Using Indirect Whole-Body Calorimetry, British Journal of Nutrition. 1989. Mar; 61(2):175-86.

accurately predict the study participants' calorie expenditure, with sleep energy expenditure used to equal basal metabolic rate, it all just clicked. I'm sure you are itching to learn the inner workings of this hack, so let's discuss the heart rate monitors I recommend.

Two of the most noted heart rate monitors on the market today are the Fitbit and the BodyBugg by bodymedia. I use Bodymedia, but both are good for our purposes. What sets these HRM's apart from others is the ability to measure energy output through changes in skin temperature. Other calorie counters, such as the Nike+ Fuelband, can't measure doing both light activity and lifting workouts effectively, since those devices don't know the difference between picking up a feather or an Olympic barbell.

As for the food scale, almost any food scale will do. I have a food scale with a 5-pound limit and I've never needed it to go higher. You probably wouldn't want to get a scale with lower weighing capabilities than 5 pounds if you plan to measure food on a plate and tare out each item. Taring just means bringing the scale back to 0 before adding a new item.

If you do not already own any of these items, I was able to get special deals for my readers. Simply visit www.thighgaphack.com/deals to take advantage of the promotion. In the interest of full disclosure, I get a small referral fee if you decide to buy, but you should know I wouldn't recommend a product I didn't truly believe in. You are also free to purchase different products.

You are required to wear the heart rate monitor all day, every day. The only time you are permitted to take the monitor off is when you are showering. I can hear your moans and groans now, but it won't be forever! Generally, it takes only three weeks to develop a habit, so after that time your new hunger patterns should be solidified. What follows below is a detailed example of how one would use this protocol.

Again, the easiest way to implement Hunger Training™ is with a heart rate monitor that will display how many calories you have burned on a screen or watch on a minute-by-minute basis.

First, take your body weight and multiply it by 10 - 12. Use 10 if you want faster weight loss, 11 for moderate weight loss, and 12 for slower weight loss. This is the amount of calories you will be eating per day. Does this mean that you can never deviate? No, some days you can eat 10x, while others days you will eat 11x or 12x. In fact, doing so would mirror another hack, calorie cycling, that we cover in great detail later on. Once you arrive at your figure, you will need to keep it in mind so that you do not continue to eat once it has been reached.

Upon awakening, you will be required to reset your HRM and not eat until it has shown a sizeable calorie burn. The calories of your first meal will depend on this number (it cannot exceed it), and determine the other times you should eat as well as the amount of calories per subsequent meal according to how much you have burned.

For example, a 100-pound woman determines she needs to eat 1200 calories for the day (slower weight loss). Upon waking she resets her HRM. She eats a maximum 400-Calorie breakfast at 11am when her HRM says she has burned 400 calories. Once her HRM shows another 400-Calorie burn, she will be free to eat up to 400 calories again. If she wants to speed things up she'll be more active.

To continue our example, she may burn 400 calories in 3 hours (2pm), at which point she has another 400 Calorie meal. She then burns that 400 calories after 5 hours and eats her last meal consisting of 400 calories at 7pm. Eating in this retroactive manner ensure her body has used up the energy provided by every meal before being supplied more food, plus the desired deficit has been accounted for by using the multiple of 12 to determine slow weight loss.

There's one more element to Hunger Training™ that I thought I'd save for last so that it wouldn't get lost in the shuffle. This last rule was put in place to prevent you from eating too much, and it is: Do not go to bed before you have burned off all the calories from your last meal. Thus, if you know that you want to go to sleep at 11pm and it'll take approximately 4 hours to burn off your 400-Calorie meal, make sure you stop eating at 7pm. When you're sleeping and feel hungry, your body will turn to its fat stores.

ALTERNATIVE HUNGER TRAINING™ PROTOCOL

For those of you who are unable to get a HRM and still want to try Hunger Training™, there is another, albeit less precise, way to do it. First, determine how many calories you burn per day at rest by adding your basal metabolic rate to the amount of calories you burn via exercise associated thermogenesis or EAT (calorie burned through exercise), and non-exercise activity thermogenesis or NEAT (calories burned from your every day activities).

Once you accomplish this you can tell roughly how many calories your body burns per hour by dividing your overall calories by twenty-four. Simply follow the rest of the protocol that outlines retroactively eating once the appropriate amount of calories have been burned.

There are a few ways to calculate your BMR, NEAT and EAT. Much like the various tests and tools we covered above to calculate your body fat, accuracy will vary. BMR is measured using oxygen consumed or using a metabolic chamber and is the precursor to figuring out your Total Daily Energy Expenditure (TDEE).

ONLINE CALCULATORS

The most accessible tool for most individuals will be an online calculator, including not only specific "BMR online calculators", but also free food logging software and weight loss websites that seek to assist you in your target calorie intake. They are going to give you a very rough estimate that can be close to your real numbers or completely miss the mark, with most missing the mark. An excellent and accurate online calculator (according to those who have compared the results of official tests to this online calculator) is the intermittent fasting calculator. This calculator is free of charge and can be found by searching for "intermittent fasting calculator" in google.com or by visiting www.1percentedge.com/ifcalc/. It's one of the rare online calculators that takes your lean body fat into account.

Despite the great reviews for the Intermittent Fasting Calculator, I'd strongly encourage you to try other calculators out as well. Having figures from multiple calculators will give you an idea of what's going on inside your body. Be aware that many will grossly overestimate, rather than underestimate, your TDEE. Thus, it is safer to assume the lowest numbers will be the closest to being correct.

More cautionary advice for using online calculators is to make sure you input the proper variables for your activity level. The choices will normally be sedentary, lightly active, mildly/moderately active, very active, etc. This is one of the main variables in the formula for arriving at your final numbers. Thus, choosing the appropriate option is key.

If you work out a few times per week, chances are you will want to mark down leading a mildly active or active lifestyle, however I would advise you to select sedentary instead. Imagine two individuals working out 4 times per week, but someone giving 100% every workout having the same numbers as someone who barely breaks a sweat during their workout. Clearly, both individuals would be at a disadvantage when it comes to how many calories they can consume if they go with those numbers that do not truly reflect their energy expenditure.

Besides this fact, the reality is most people lead very sedentary lives outside of the few times they exercise. Our jobs require us to sit around all day, and when we get home, we aren't suddenly becoming very active. By the way, walking to get to and from the couch or kitchen, or to the train/bus hardly counts as an active lifestyle! The intensity level of your walk is probably not resulting in huge Calories being burned, and most Americans simply are not walking enough to do anything for weight loss. If you don't believe me, buy a pedometer and prepared to be shocked.

Another factor against choosing any other activity level beside sedentary, is to consider the numbers are an average of how many Calories you burn spread out over the week. This would be fine if each day and every time you worked out, you burned the same number of Calories, but you don't.

A better approach is to make a conservative estimate towards your calories burned whenever you exercise. There are online programs where you can plug in your activity, length and intensity of workout, and age/weight/etc. and the program will spit out how many calories you've burned. Account for net calories burned (the amount of calories you would have burned in the same amount of time) by subtracting this number from your workout calories burned, and feel free to use this final number to gauge when to eat your next meal on the Hunger Training Protocol™.

If you want to get even more accurate than an online calculator and cannot use the heart rate monitors I recommend in the original Hunger Training Protocol™, consider The Metabolic Analyzer test. It accurately calculates the number of Calories you would burn if you were to be at rest for 24 hours. This is called your Resting Metabolic Rate (RMR) or your maintenance Calories. The Metabolic Analyzer is an indirect calculator and is considered to be the gold standard for calculating maintenance Calories as it can accurately calculate the Calories burned during a day for an individual without estimates or predictions.

The test takes only 10-15 minutes to complete. But the results and the interpretation of the results might take almost 45 minutes. The test involves breathing through a mouthpiece for 10-15 minutes. The cost can range from as little as $15 and is administered at numerous universities.

STRATEGIC FASTING

The next fat loss hack has been very successful in helping both women and men shed unwanted body fat. Fasting is generally perceived as not eating for a day or multiple days for religious purposes. We also associate fasting with starving yourself and being extremely hard. Intermittent fasting means that you literally fast intermittently (not all the time). It is based on the premise that by cutting out one meal a day (e.g. breakfast) or a full day of meals where you fast for 24 hours, you create a caloric deficit while allowing for a longer fat burning period.

Many people scoff at fasting and think it is abnormal, unnecessary or even dangerous, however before electricity and diners that stayed open 24/7, humans used to spend a long stretch every night without food passing our lips. Staying up and eating late is a very recent phenomenon in human history, so our metabolisms are actually hardwired to expect a nightly fast, which is a key time for your body to burn fat.

In fact, new studies reveal that to burn the most fat, you need to go at least twelve hours without eating (e.g.- 8 p.m. to 8 a.m. or 9 a.m. to 9 p.m.), so it's smart to time your calorie intake accordingly. On top of intermittent fasting providing a prime fat burning period, it is an excellent way to restrict Calories or prevent overeating, thus resulting in impressive fat loss. For instance, there is only so much you can eat without feeling uncomfortable and stuffed in an eight-hour eating window. If you are not permitted to eat after 8pm, as an example, there is a great chance that you will be able to adhere to your Calorie goals.

My preferred method of intermittent fasting is one where you eat in an eight-hour to ten-hour window and fast for anywhere from sixteen to fourteen hours (typically over night while you are sleeping), with sixteen hours being my individual sweet spot. There have also been studies and accounts that support many women finding the fourteen-hour fasting or ten-hour feeding period to work the best.

Either way, restricting food to a window can increase weight loss. In one study carried out by biologist Satchidananda Panda and colleagues at Salk's Regulatory Biology Laboratory, mice were fed a high-fat, high-calorie diet with one group given access to food both day and night, while the other group had access for only eight hours at night (the most active period for mice). In human terms, this would mean eating only for 8 hours during the day.

Despite consuming the same amount of calories, mice that had access to food for only eight hours stayed lean and did not develop health problems like high blood sugar or chronic inflammation. They even had improved endurance motor coordination on the exercise wheel. The all-day access group became obese and was plagued with health problems. The researchers concluded, "[Time-restricted feeding] is a non-pharmacological strategy against obesity and associated diseases."

Whether you decide to do a twelve-hour, fourteen-hour, sixteen-hour or longer fast, chances are you will be skipping breakfast as most intermittent fasters do. When I mention intermittent fasting to others I get the crazy looks and protests against skipping breakfast. The idea of breakfast, which is a relatively new concept, has been so ingrained in our every day routine that you are probably also thinking you wouldn't survive the day without a bowl of cereal the first thing in the morning.

As a quick aside, cereal is nothing but candy, and sugar in your system completely stumps your fat loss goals (as we will soon explore), so getting rid of cereals from your diet is one of the best things you could do if you're trying to get a thigh gap. For a great all natural cereal alternative search "cereal recipe" on The Feminine Contour Blog at www.thefemininecontour.com

Consider the fact that mankind didn't always have access to food upon awakening and they were able to function. Additionally, some children and adults can't eat breakfast in the morning without feeling queasy and go about their morning perfectly fine without it. They simply have no appetite. If you eat breakfast at 7:30am every morning, your body will come to expect it will be fed around that time and you will feel "hungry" out of habit.

The fact is people may "feel" hungry the first thing in the morning because their ghrelin (hunger hormone) has been entrained for that eating pattern. Our bodies get used to patterns and habits we form and respond accordingly. The more in depth explanation is Ghrelin secretion in your body happens on a schedule based on your eating schedule. In other words, the more often you eat, the more often you produce ghrelin, and the more often you want to eat. It has nothing to do with necessity for nutrients.

If you were to switch to eating twice a day (and I'm not suggesting you do), after several days or maybe a week, your hormones would adjust and you'd no longer get hungry on your old eating schedule. That's how we are able to retrain your hunger with the Hunger Training Protocol™ outlined in this book. The same applies to intermittent fasting. If you were to feed for a 10 to 6 hour window and fast for a 14 – 18 hour window every day for a week, you would similarly adjust and not feel hunger outside of those times.

Breaking the Fast

When it comes time to break the fast, eat half a grapefruit with coffee/tea an hour before your first meal. Whenever you eat something with calories, your metabolism has to increase momentarily to process incoming calories, but the net effect of grapefruit is that of a fat burner. The reason you should take it before breaking the fast is because grapefruit has carbohydrates but doesn't stimulate insulin like most other carbohydrate foods. Not to mention the stuff in grapefruit (naringen) can possibly make caffeine work better.

ZIG-ZAG CALORIE SHIFTING

Calorie cycling, which is also known as zig-zag cycling and sometimes even called carb cycling is next up on our list of fat loss hacks. However, it is imperative to note there is a marked difference between calorie cycling and carb cycling, although these terms are often used interchangeably. My preferred method for burning stubborn thigh fat is calorie cycling and I'll explain why.

The way calorie cycling works is by taking a weekly sum approach for the amount of Calories you consume, where some days you eat higher Calories and other days you eat lower Calories, as long as you do not go over your weekly calorie maximum for weight loss. The premise behind calorie cycling is that continually switching up the amount of Calories we intake on a daily basis prevents homeostasis from occurring with your metabolism, thus maximizing fat burn.

Broken down a bit further, your metabolism will try to adjust to the amount of Calories or energy you provide it with over time.

So, when you eat less over a consistent period, your body adjusts by burning less. On the contrary, your metabolism rises slightly when you provide it with more Calories on a consistent basis.

Your metabolism also goes up with more food intake thanks to something called the Thermic Effect of feeding (TEF) as you expend energy to break down, digest, absorb, and utilize the food. However, just in case you may be thinking you should start eating more often to milk this effect for all its worth, I should note here that TEF is determined by your total energy intake. It won't increase simply by eating more often or decrease by eating less often. You'll burn a set number based on total calories.

What do you do with that information? Well, when you alternate between switching your caloric intake from a higher amount for a few days, where you get your metabolism revving, to considerably eating less the next day or so, your metabolism is still operating at that higher level and you burn more Calories than you normally would had you eaten lower calories consecutively (your metabolism would have slowed to compensate for the lessened fuel). Thus, you are effectively able to trick your body into burning more calories and have days where you can eat heartily.

Of course, if you continue eating a low amount of Calories, your metabolism will undoubtedly adjust downward again, so the cycle continues (hence the name Calorie Cycling) until you reach your goal weight or goal body composition and switch to eating at a maintenance level.

Carb cycling differs in that you are making sure to eat more carbs on certain days than on others, which I do not condone for our purposes. Carb cycling is also known in the bodybuilding world as carb back loading and is used as a means for making muscle gains while remaining lean.

It requires heavy lifting a few hours before (and sometimes after) eating a high carb meal, as the carb load provides energy to complete more intense workouts. Besides many proponents of this technique opting for calorie dense foods filled with simple sugars like cake, doughnuts, pizza and the like to meet their carb requirements, carbs indirectly cause increased activity in the fat suppressing receptors in the thighs (alpha adrenergic receptors abundant in the subcutaneous fat of the female lower body) by releasing insulin.

Another thing to keep in mind is anecdotally, many have been able to remain the same "weight" while seeing more muscle definition and increasing inches in circumference on arms, chest and legs via carb cycling, so unless you want to gain inches on your legs and thighs, stay away.

With carb cycling, on the days which you eat more carbs, you will subsequently burn less fat and more carbs which is the last thing we want. Becoming fat adapted by training your body to primarily burn fat as opposed to glycogen later is a much better idea.

Scratching your head yet? It's quite simple actually. When you consume carbohydrates, they are rapidly broken down into glucose (sugar) in the body. Your body works hard to maintain blood concentrations of various nutrients and chemicals and as a result releases insulin into your blood stream. Insulin tells your cells to absorb the sugar out of the blood as sugar and any other nutrient must be carefully regulated and removed quickly if it gets too high. It also tells your fat cells not to release any fat to burn because there are already carbs in the blood to burn.

Since your body will burn carbs before stored fat, naturally the less carbs your body has to burn through before turning to fat and stored fat cells, the quicker and higher your weight loss will be. To put it plainly, the less carbs present, the more fat burned. This is what is called being fat adapted.

Another major differentiator between carb cycling and calorie cycling is that with carb cycling, you may be eating the exact same amount of Calories every day and simply increasing and decreasing the carb amounts, which means you inversely increase or decrease the protein/fat content of your foods.

With calorie cycling, you are specifically increasing and decreasing the amount of Calories consumed on various days. The difference in overall Calories between these two methods can add up and make a huge impact on your weight loss as Calories in and Calories out will always determine the amount of fat you burn and weight you lose.

Here is a straightforward example to illustrate my point:

Carb Cycling

Let's say you consume 1500 Calories per day for a total of 10,500 Calories per week. You shift the amount of carbs you consume on workout days and non workout days and may be able to work out harder on workout days given carbs are a source of energy, however your body will be doing just that – burning carbs or glycogen because it has plenty of it in the form of your higher carbs. We don't want this.

Instead, we want the body to turn to your fat for energy, which it can only do if there is not a lot of glycogen stores in the first place. On top of this, your metabolism adjusts to this predictable amount of daily energy input so that it is more likely that you will maintain your current weight of plateau as opposed to losing fat/weight.

Calorie Cycling

You may consume 1200 Calories on 3 non-workout days in which you don't require as much energy, and 1500 Calories on 4 workout days when you do, resulting in a total of 9600. That's a difference of 900 Calories as it compares to our previous carb cycling example above. Since it takes 3500 Calories to lose one pound of fat, you would lose an additional pound per month, on top of the deficit you would have already been creating with your caloric intake.

It gets even better. The days when your overall Calories are higher, your metabolism will rise to adjust to the higher caloric input. When you then suddenly switch to a lower calorie day, it takes a few days for your metabolism to adjust to that new setting. So what you get is the benefit of a higher metabolism burning through your fat stores thus meeting our objective of manipulating your metabolism in your favor.

To summarize, calorie cycling or calorie shifting means to deliberately eat much fewer Calories on certain days and more Calories on other days to take advantage of an increased metabolism that results in higher calorie days, thus burning more fat than you would otherwise on lower calorie days. It may all sound a bit complicated, but calorie cycling is a highly effective and recommended technique you can use to target the stubborn body fat on your hips and thighs.

Now that you know the major distinction between calorie and carb cycling as well as how it works, let's turn to how go about implementing calorie cycling the proper way.

CALORIE CYCLING PROTOCOL

The first part of Calorie Cycling requires you to figure out the total amount of Calories you will be able to consume for the entire week. This is the maximum number of Calories you are able to safely eat in order to stay in a calorie deficit and lose between one and two pounds of weight per week. If your starting weight is lower, the smaller your calorie deficit should be so that you don't have to restrict calories to the point of feeling constantly hungry.

As discussed in a previous chapter, one pound of fat is equal to approximately 3500 Calories; therefore if you have a caloric deficit of about 500 Calories per day, over the course of seven days you would have eaten at a deficit of 3500 Calories, which would translate to a one-pound loss on your scale. The standard guideline in the fitness industry is to take 20 – 30% of your total daily energy expenditure to come up with your calorie deficit. For example, if you expend 2,000 Calories of energy, 20% of 2000 would be 400, thus you would eat 1600 Calories for a daily deficit of 400. After about 8 or 9 days of such a deficit you would lose one pound of fat, as 3500/400 = 8.75.

CRUNCHING THE NUMBERS

To get to the maximum number of Calories you will be able to eat per day and week, we must calculate or get a close estimate of your BMR and TDEE, which can be found in the Alternate Hunger Training Protocol™ section. We will then figure out the appropriate deficit to meet your required weekly weight loss goals and finally, come up with the weekly Calories.

For example, let's say that your base metabolic rate is 1200 Calories, you burn 700 additional Calories through engaging in your day to day activities and exercise and you want to lose one pound of fat or end up with a deficit of 3500 food Calories over the course of the week. Expending 1900 Calories of energy per day (your BMR + TDEE), less 500 Calories per day (because 500 Calories over seven days will equal 3500 Calories) will leave you with a balance of 1400 Calories per day. 1400 Calories per day over the course of 7 days will give you with a total weekly sum of 9800 Calories that may be consumed.

Thus, for the purposes of calorie cycling, as long as you do not go above 9800 Calories per week, you will be able to eat more or less than 1400 Calories on a daily basis. In other words, instead of focusing on limiting your Calories at 1400 per day to reach 9800 Calories for the week, your daily Calories could look something more like this: 1,200, 1400, 1400, 1200, 1600, 1200, 1800. Notice, if you add all the numbers up you still reach 9800 Calories.

To iterate, if you choose to use an online calculator over a high quality heart rate monitor, select sedentary for your activity level to determine your starter TDEE every day. Add a conservative estimate of calories (taking into account the net calorie effect) for the specific workout you do that day for your overall TDEE. This means your TDEE will be fluctuating daily, as it should.

It is important to note here, your basal metabolic rate will change every time you lose 5 to 10 pounds, so your BMR will need to be re-evaluated and re-calculated periodically as you will not need as much energy to carry less body weight around. Subsequently, you will have to adjust your calorie intake or energy expenditure to meet your fitness/weight loss goals.

Lastly, in order for Calorie Cycling to work even faster and more effectively, engage in more intense exercise on the higher Calorie days and either rest or do lighter exercises such as walking or low intensity steady state cardio on the lower Calorie days.

HACK TIP

CALCULATING CALORIES BURNED

Do not depend on the numbers given to you by workout machines, as they are notorious for overestimating your energy expenditure. Just how off are the Calories burned numbers given by machines? The University of California at San Francisco's Human Performance Center, which specializes in physiological analysis, uses a VO2 test to track fat burning down to the last calorie. The test works by measuring the maximum capacity of an individual's breathing while exercising.

The VO2 analyzer assesses a user's Calories lost during exercise by tracking breathing patterns. First, the user puts on headgear similar to a scuba mask and snorkel. The snorkel is attached to a long tube that is hooked into the VO2 analyzer. Finally, the analyzer records the user's breathing pattern as he or she inhales and exhales during exercise. Depending on the quality of breathing, the VO2 analyzer calculates how hard the user is working and combines that data with the user's body stats: height, weight, age, and body fat. The VO2 analyzer can then compute how many Calories are burned during the exercise.

GMA technology contributor Becky Worley used the VO2 test on a treadmill, stationary bike, stair climber, elliptical machine and fitness watches, each for five minutes. In each case, according to the VO2 test, the number of Calories burned was overestimated, with an overestimation of 19% by machines and

28% percent by watches on average. The detailed breakdown of the individual machines were as follows[6]:

Treadmill: Overestimated Calories burnt by 13%

Stationary Bike: Overestimated Calories burnt by 7%

Stair Climber: Overestimated Calories burnt by 12%

Elliptical: Overestimated Calories burnt by 42%

That last percentage was not a typo. Ladies, can you imagine basing your daily calorie intakes on an overestimation of 42%! Instead of taking in 1500 Calories you actually need, you'd end up with an extra 630 Calories per day, and gain 1 pound every 5 or 6 days (3500 divided by 650). If you were like most people, you'd blame the weight gain on a broken metabolism or something else equally silly and insignificant since you'd be convinced you were doing everything right.

———————————

[6] abcnews.go.com/GMA/Weekend/exercise-calorie-counters-work/story?id=9966500#.UWle9I479Vx

Avoid the above scenario by investing in the most accurate heart rate monitor on the market. At the moment Polar, Mio Alpha and Bodymedia appear to be the market leaders, but you can be sure to find the most updated reviews and referrals by visiting www.thighgaphack.com/resources.

You may also assume the numbers given to you by many devices are going to skew up, so take preventative measures by rounding your readings down by 10%. A final way to try to get as close to your calories burned during exercise is to plug your stats into online programs and formulas that provide calories burned per exercise and take the average or lowest number spit out. Select programs and calculators that take stats such as height, weight, age, and body measurements into consideration to get more reliable figures.

GROSS VS NET CALORIES

As previously mentioned, do remember to distinguish between whether your calories burned are representative of gross or net calories burned. Fitness equipment, heart rate monitors and the like do not automatically do the calculation for you and not knowing the difference between gross and net Calories is a crucial misstep that result in overestimation of Calories burned.

Since you will actually be determining how many Calories you can eat given these numbers, every detail counts. Net calorie burn, for any given physical activity, is the amount of calories burned only to perform the physical activity, and no more. Net calories is simply figuring out how many calories you would have burned during the time you worked out and subtracting it from the calories actually burned during physical exercise.

Gross calorie burn is the absolute total amount of Calories burned while performing any given activity. It includes the Calories that your body burned specifically to perform the activity itself, plus the additional Calories burned throughout the duration of the physical activity that your body must continually burn at all times to digest food, keep tissues alive, and support the function of vital organs. As opposed to gross calorie burn, net calorie burn does not include Calories burned to support your RMR.[7]

---

[7] Shapesense - www.shapesense.com/fitness-exercise/articles/net-versus-

Typical calorie burn calculators, including those usually built into treadmills, stair climbers, bikes, elliptical machines, etc., provide gross calorie burn estimates, but some calculators provide net calorie burn estimates. As long as you know what numbers you're working with, you can use either one.

FAT FREEZE

Thermogenesis is the process of heat production in mammals. Cold Thermogenesis is heat production stimulated by exposure to cold temperatures.

One study found that decreased thermogenesis may in itself be causative of obesity; correspondingly, 'induced' thermogenesis counteracts obesity (even without dietary intervention). Thus, activation of thermogenesis is an anti-obesity tool irrespective of whether it is accomplished by artificial uncoupling, exercise, shivering, or recruitment and activation of brown adipose tissue. The latter would seem to be the more physiological, and the more comfortable, of these means of promoting thermogenesis.[8]

---

[8] journals.cambridge.org/produc...textid=6406180

The magic behind CT is in activation of BAT (brown fat) and Uncoupling Proteins. BAT burns calories to create heat, thanks to a little guy called uncoupling protein-1 (UCP-1) which allows the mitochondria to burn through fuel at alarming rates. Uncoupling Proteins (UCP-1) create a huge impact on metabolism far longer than the time exposed to cold.

Anything you can do to increase your exposure to cold temperatures will increase your metabolism. This is because your body wants to maintain it's internal temperature around 98.6 degree Fahrenheit. When it senses cold, it will increase the rate of cellular activity to keep the core temperature optimal for survival.

Why is activating BAT a good thing? For starters, BAT acts as a natural heating system and contains loads of mitochondria, miniature power stations, which among other things can 'burn' fat. In doing this, they normally generate a voltage similar to that of a battery, which then provides energy for cellular processes. However, the mitochondria of brown fat cells have a short circuit. They go full steam ahead all the time. The energy released when the fat is broken down is released as heat.

Babies are born with lots of BAT; they would get cold very quickly without this mechanism. When our core temperature starts to drop, the thermostat kicks the furnace on and we heat up the core and to a lesser degree, the rest of our body.

It was previously thought that BAT was lost with age but recent findings have showed that adults have a deposit of BAT in the neck, supraclavicular region, chest and abdomen under PET-CT scans only after exposure to mild cold.[9] If we have a need for it, we'd have more though and one such reason is chronic exposure to cold.

It is widely shown that people with lots of BAT are lean, while obese people have relatively little BAT. Women are also twice as likely as men to have significant amounts of active brown fat — perhaps because with less muscle mass, they need brown fat to stay warm.

---

[9] www.nejm.org/doi/pdf/10.1056/NEJMoa0808718

BAT can be recruited from White Adipose Tissue, it is then called BRITE (brown from white). In other words, brown fat actually uses regular fat from the rest of the body to fuel itself. Unlike white fat, which stores energy, chestnut-colored brown fat burns it. This happens seasonally in almost everybody and is tied to light cycles and temperature, though more to light cycles.

HOW TO DO IT

It is recommended that to ease into cold water therapy, you should do face dunks, where you fill a basin with ice cold water (add ice if your tap water doesn't get cold enough) and simply dunk your face until you can't bear it anymore, for most about 20 seconds. Repeat this 3 to 5 times. Your body will think you fell into cold water and will prepare you for the more vigorous methods. This alone won't get the job done, but a side benefit is that the skin on your face will look amazing!

To activate the BAT there are a few things you can and should do. You can take a cold shower for at least 30 seconds and let it run over your shoulders, neck and back, building up the minutes you expose yourself to the cold water over time.

Alternatively, you could use an ice pack or take cold baths for 20 minutes or more depending on your tolerance level. Simply fill a gallon size plastic bag half full with ice cubes and a little water, and move the ice pack around when it starts to turn your skin red (2-3 minutes). You can easily get an hour out of an ice pack like this. Many have been known to place the packs around the neck (above the collarbone), chest and collarbones as well as the abdomen and the thighs.

You could also soak your feet in 45-degree water as doing so for 5 minutes has been shown on Pet scan studies to activate BAT. The studies suggest 'winter' isn't sensed until you are exposed to approximately 50 degrees Fahrenheit. You can do one method or all three as well as find other way to expose yourself to the cold more often. The goal is to give your body a reason to react to the cold. As far as how long you should be cold, the best way to activate BAT is to remain as long as you can in the temperature zone between "getting goosebumps" and "shivering". Once you start shivering the BAT turns off, as the muscles take over warming the body, so if you are shivering, back off - it's too cold!

The above should be done on an empty stomach because you will find yourself hungry once you warm back up as your body tries to put you back to zero after such a large dumping of thermodynamic heat (stored energy, not temperature). Be sure to plan for this feeling of hunger by fixing a large, calorie-restricted meal (avoid calorie dense foods) ahead of time.

There are those who say that doing this protocol will not work, but research, plus anecdotal evidence from those who have tried cold therapy, supports the effects are real.

A team led by Sven Enerbäck, a medical geneticist at the University of Gothenburg in Sweden, found that when subjects spent 2 hours in a cold room wearing thin clothing and intermittently soaking their feet in ice water, their brown fat burned 15 times more energy than it did at room temperature. One subject had enough brown fat to lose 8 to 9 pounds per year. Dutch researchers found active brown fat in 23 out of 24 subjects when they were cold, but not when they were warm. Researchers estimate that just 2 ounces of active brown fat could burn 300 to 500 calories a day.

Here's one final tidbit of good news: the more BAT is active, the more it grows and the more BAT you have, the hotter your metabolism will run. Makes you want to stop reading right now and ice your way through the rest of this book right? I completely approve! Just remember that while cold therapy will give you a boost in metabolism and calorie burn, it's not a cure all for giving us the contoured bodies we are after.

HACK TIP

Don't Just Drink Water

You've heard about drinking 8 cups of water a day, but if you want to increase your metabolism and burn more calories you'd be better off drinking ice cold water. Drinking ice water all day is an excellent way to increase your metabolism to the tune of 200-300 extra calories burned per day. Use finely crushed ice and swallow the ice along with the water

N. E. A. T

There are things some people naturally have that give them a unique advantage when it comes to staying thin. To name a few, possessing great genes, having a naturally slender build or a ridiculously fast metabolism, being taller (thus burning more calories and requiring more food), cannot be copied, but one fact that is largely responsible for many a thin person's lithe figure can be emulated. That is Non Exercise Activity Thermogenesis or NEAT.

NEAT is precisely what it sounds like; the energy expended for everything we do that is not sleeping, eating or sports-like exercise. NEAT could burn up to 1000 extra calories per day when properly incorporated throughout the day. As previously mentioned in the section on calculating your BMR using online calculators, most people will need to choose sedentary as their activity level because a majority of modern human beings lead sedentary lives. You can thank the remote control, elevators, microwave, dishwasher, cars, the Internet and many more technological advances and inventions for why we move less in general.

Having said that, it should come as no surprise that one study found a habit of naturally thin people is that they lead active lives outside of specific exercise activity[10]. You may know a person or two like this who can't keep still, is constantly on the move and/or fidgeting, or involved in a lot of recreational activities and hobbies (e.g. hiking or dancing). Of course, one aspect of this equation is that these individuals do not overcompensate for their increased activity be overeating or treating themselves for all of the activity they do, as far too many people who exercise fall victim to doing.

You, too, can reap the benefits of non-exercise activity thermogenesis by hacking your sedentary tendencies. The following hacks are ways to force yourself to be more active outside of exercise. Start using them and see the difference.

WEAR A PEDOMETER

---

[10] Levine JA et. al. Role of nonexercise activity thermogenesis in resistance to fat gain in humans. Science. (1999) Jan 8;283(5399):212-4.

Pedometers are relatively cheap beeper-sized devices worn on the body, typically on the waist, which tracks the number of steps an individual takes each day. Set daily goals for yourself and then meet it no matter what. If the end of the day is approaching and you haven't met your step count, then you'll know it's time to go for a walk around the block. Generally, I've found that the simple act of wearing a pedometer encourages you to take more steps, especially if you log your step count somewhere visible every day (like on a paper on the refrigerator door). Enlisting others in your family or joining groups can make increasing steps competitive and fun.

PARK AWAY

I've done it, you've done it, we all do it. What's 'it'? Pull up to valet parking, circle around a parking lot or wait in the car for what seems like days on end, just to get the closest parking space possible to your destination. Use these opportunities to rack up NEAT points, and in some instances save a ton of time, by parking further away and walking just a little bit longer to get to your destination.

TAKE THE STAIRS

No Doubt you've heard this advice before, but it's worth repeating. If I had a dollar for every time I've seen someone wait for an elevator up or down one single floor in my life, I'd be on the cover of Forbes. If you want to save time and get more NEAT in, challenge yourself to take the stairs going down every time! Walking down stairs hardly requires any exertion. Eventually, you want to adapt this habit when walking up the stairs as well, but to start off it is totally fine to take the stairs up as many flights as possible and then switch to an elevator or escalator.

TAKE A NEAT INVENTORY

Most modern inventions since the wheel have served to reduce NEAT. If you really want to take advantage of this very simple and effective hack to leaning out your body, take stock of the things you've grown accustomed to that lower your NEAT points every day. The following are just some ideas, but feel free to dedicate some brain power to figuring out things you currently use that are supposed to make your life easier, that could be an opportunity to increase your NEAT.

Vow not to use the remote control and set your television to turn off automatically every 30 minutes to force you to get up and moving (even if it's just to turn the TV back on).

Ditch the bi-weekly or monthly bulk grocery shopping trips for daily or weekly trips to the farmer's market. Buying in bulk means fewer trips to the grocery store and more easy access to food. Buying fresh food daily, or as you need it will lead to you consuming less as well as providing a great opportunity to increase NEAT. To really ramp things up, carry your groceries home.

Seek out those items that are meant to do things for you and eliminate them. Examples are the dishwasher, electronic toothbrush, bathroom tile sprays that don't require scrubbing, drive through car wash, microwave, drop off/pick up laundry services, etc. Really take stock of the things that are supposed to make life more convenient and then go back to the original way of doing that thing, which is more than likely to help raise your NEAT.

LUNCH DANCE PARTIES

Lunchtime dance parties, a daytime party for an hour, are happening in cities all across the world, and is an excellent way to fit more non-exercise activity into your life. Lunch Beat, one such party, was founded by Molly Range, who was inspired by "Fight Club," David Fincher's film about white-collar workers who form secret societies to tear one another up. There are more than 50 Lunch Beat chapters around the world, including New York. Another party series, Lunch Rocks, was started by Thomas Rudy and his wife, Amanda Tan, and draws hundreds of people per event.

Both Lunch Beach and Lunch Break charge between $10 and $15 per ticket. Despite the name, these parties take the emphasis off food and place it on dancing, so don't expect an overflowing buffet of dishes. Many also serve alcohol, but you are not required to imbibe (and I don't recommend you do) lest you spoil the advantages of your increased NEAT by ingesting liquor calories. Plus, you'll have to return to work after your lunch break, and showing up inebriated may not be the best idea.

If one of these establishments is not currently in your area, you could be the one to open a new chapter. Alternatively, taking a 30 - 45 minute dance class in the area on your lunch break would also suffice.

Part 5 – Eat Stubborn Fat Away

THE THIGH GAP DIET™

There are plenty of diets out there promising results. There are equally as many people on each of those diets, oftentimes with totally conflicting advice and claims, yielding weight and fat loss results. But which one is best for our purposes of hacking your thigh and stubborn lower body fat?

If you notice, plenty of fat loss diets, from Atkins to the Slow Carb, to the South Beach Diet, to the newest and hottest kid on the block, Paleo or Primal eating, have a lot of things in common, such as avoid sugars, highly processed foods and refined carbs. Many diets can be reduced to low carbs, moderate to high protein and moderate to high fat. Of course some diet plans out there say you can eat high fat, or high protein, or high carb or even eat all you want, but I have yet to find one that's not a gimmick that advocated doing all of the above.

Typically the dieter has to compensate for the high fat, protein or carb foods by decreasing the other macronutrients. Not surprisingly, when you have to eat less of any macronutrient or start cutting out food groups, you wind up with lower overall Calories, which is a critical component of weight loss. However, not all macronutrients are equal and some diets are harder to follow as well as sustain for this exact reason.

I recommend a mash up of the best practices from many diets that will keep you full and satiated so that you aren't always hungry and thinking about food. As a result, it will be easier to meet your lowered caloric goals and control your hormones. The dieting strategies I am about to outline should be used with hunger training, intermittent fasting and/or calorie cycling for even faster results.

If for any reason you are prevented from eating as I recommend (e.g. – fruitarians, vegetarians or raw vegans) feel free to deviate, but doing so may make adherence to the calorie deficit needed to shed fat a little harder. For those of you who find yourself in that camp, try to stick to the basic tenets of a good diet by figuring out your caloric needs (your calorie deficit) and meeting it by cutting out as much sugar and highly processed foods as you can. Take in a good amount of fiber and water throughout the day, and you should see some pretty great improvements in your fat loss and body composition over time.

DIET OVERVIEW

The best diet for lowering your body fat and achieving the thigh gap of your dreams will be low carbohydrates, high fiber, very low sugar and salt, moderate fat, moderate to high protein, high nutrition, whole foods or food that come to us by nature without a lot of preservatives, added ingredients and minimal processing, and no to low dairy.

Losing fat is such a seemingly evasive thing to do because the foods that are prevalent in our society contain too much refined carbohydrates, cheese, sugar, oil, salt and not nearly enough whole plants and protein. No one is safe, not even vegetarians or vegans. If you are vegetarian or vegan, you will need to find your protein sources somewhere besides meat, and you have to watch out for many of the imitation foods that are calorie dense as well as filled with sugar/carbs and oil.

I don't eat red meat or pork, so I completely understand and respect not wanting to consume meat or animal byproducts, but if you find yourself turning to highly processed carbs and sugary foods because you are tired of vegetables and find your choices limited, your stubborn fat won't be doing much budging.

LOW CARBOHYDRATES

You've heard the success stories of those who follow the Atkins Diet™, made famous for its low carb, high protein content. You have probably also heard of the numerous criticisms of the diet as well. Some have claimed that it is incredibly difficult to sustain a low carb diet due to the dearth of yummy high carb foods that are available to us, but I find this to be a cop out. No one ever says it is incredibly difficult to sustain a drug free life due to the dearth of drugs that are around us, right? The point is, if you know something is bad for you, regardless of whether your co-workers are always ordering pizza or your friends are always baking chocolate cakes, you don't consume those things and you certainly don't seek them out.

Let me back up a little bit and start at the beginning. What are carbs, why do they get such a bad rep and why are they also so successful in helping people lose weight? I'll answer these questions and tell you why I strongly recommend you go the low carb route to accomplish your goal of thinner thighs.

Carbs are classified as starches and sugars, and make up the essence of bread, cereal, corn, potatoes, cookies, pasta, fruit, juice, candy, beer, and sweetened drinks —basically anything that isn't protein or fat. According to USDA dietary recommendations, they are not only healthy but are supposed to make up the majority of the food we eat (45 to 65 percent of all Calories). Of course, these guidelines were established in the 1970s and have since been accompanied by an explosion of obesity and diabetes. The advice came about as early nutrition scientists rallied around the misguided maxim that eating too much fat makes you fat, despite science never bearing this to be true. More than likely, the proclamation of carbs being a necessary part of the food pyramid probably had everything to do with it being the one nutrient that is cheap and amenable to commercial mass production.

However, as a pair of Harvard doctors (one an endocrinologist and one an epidemiologist) wrote in the Journal of the

American Medical Association, carbohydrates are "a nutrient for which humans have no absolute requirement." What we now know to be true is that at the center of the obesity universe lie carbohydrates, not fat. Still, the fabric of many attitudes remains unchanged toward food to this day because of this pre-Galilean view of nutrition.

One completely false criticism that seems to have permeated the brains of the mass public is that low carb diets cause people to become lethargic and skip workouts because carbohydrates are a main source of energy that the body and the brain needs. Of course, the people who say this fail to realize that the body can also use stored body fat as energy and in fact, this is exactly what we want to have happen when you are trying to lose stubborn fat. It's how you sleep through the night without eating for eight hours. The body is perfectly happy to make fuel out of protein, leafy green vegetables, and the animal fat you're burning.

Granted, it does take a small period of time to adjust to burning fat for fuel (being fat adapted), but your workouts can be just as good when your body turns to its fat stores for energy instead of carbohydrates, and we have already covered the abundance of fat being carried around on our bodies. The excess fat, combined with the foods we always have access to, is enough to give us lasting energy for a very long time!

Another misconception about low carb diets is that they do not lead to true fat loss and instead only cause water loss. The rapid weight loss that low-carb dieters experience is said to be simply due to water weight being shed. While it is partially true that giving up carbs will result in quick weight loss due to the amount of water carbohydrates store, which is pretty awesome in my opinion, once the carbs are out of the system and the individual continues to limit carb intake, fat loss becomes inevitable.

The truth about carbs is, when stacked up against the competition, carbohydrates have the largest impact on insulin secretion. In comparison, protein has the second greatest and fat has little to no impact on insulin secretion. All that really means is what I have been stressing all along, and what I will continue to stress so that you can see what is standing between you and your thigh gap. Carbohydrates promote fat storage by providing the materials (glycerol), as well as the hormonal environment (insulin) for fat storage.

As a quick review of why we aren't such big fans of high levels of insulin, it signals the body to stop burning fat (even in a deficit) and promotes fat storage. Carbohydrates signal your body to release insulin to get the toxic sugars out of the blood stream and into the muscles. Some people are also insulin resistant, which means their bodies get so used to frequent sugars and insulin spikes that it stops responding appropriately to the spikes resulting in the body producing even more insulin to get the job done. Not good.

As long as that insulin is in your system, you can kiss your fat burning dreams good-bye, so limiting the amount of carbohydrates and sugars you intake is absolutely necessary for our purposes.

If you thought that was all there is to it, think again. The evidence against carbohydrates and sugars abound. Studies also suggest that those fast burning carbohydrates that give you a great rush lead to cravings in your brain and intrusive thoughts when you go too long without a fix.

In other words, simple carbohydrates are addictive, potentially more so than cocaine! But unlike cocaine, carbs are cheap, easy to get your hands on and does more than rewire your neurological system; it will short-circuit your body. Not only will a diet flush with carbohydrates reprogram your metabolism, locking your food away as unburnable fat, when you get hungry again (which will be shortly after your carb or sugar filled meal) you won't crave anything but more of the same food that started you down the path to dependency. On the contrary, if you eat a low processed carb diet, you are able to remain satiated between meals, because the body will take longer to break down the foods you give it.

The next logical question then is what is a low carb diet and how much should you limit your carbohydrate intake to prevent insulin spikes from occurring and blocking your fat loss attempts?

Clearly, not all carbohydrates are created the same. After all, I recommend you get plenty of vegetables and fiber, both of which translate to some carb intake. The acceptable sources of such carbohydrates are complex carbohydrates found in green, leafy, fibrous vegetables/greens and root vegetables such as sweet potato. Some diets, like Atkins™, recommend limiting net, not total, carb intake from 15 to 20 grams a day during a two-week induction phase and subsequent weekly phases to bring about ketosis, which metabolizes stored fat.

The idea behind Atkins™ is you get to slowly reintroduce complex carbohydrates back into the diet, so that ultimately you gain control over insulin (the problem not being insulin itself, but too much insulin). The two-week induction phase acts as the detox period to kick your simple carb addiction. When you introduce back complex carbs, insulin is raised more gradually and you are less likely to experience an increased appetite. Complex carbs are also likely to contain vitamins and other important nutrients. Finally, unlike simple carbs, this type of carb will not result in the body rushing to pack away all the sugars in your blood into your cells, resulting in low-blood sugar and an increased appetite.

CARB HACK TIPS

CURBING INSUILIN SPIKES

You can avoid insulin spikes by eating foods with a low Glycemic index or GI rating. Foods and their GI scores can be found by entering "glycemic index of foods" in the search tab at www.pennmedicine.org/

PAIRING FOODS

Another method is to never eat carbs by themselves. If you eat a bit of fat and protein with your carbs there is less of a chance of a large spike in insulin.

CARB-HEAVY FUNCTIONS

Once you change your diet, get ready to become increasingly aware of the abundance of processed carb heavy foods and lack of healthier options available at most functions and events. Someone trying to stick to a low-processed carb diet is usually severely limited in what he or she can eat and this presents the prime opportunity to fall off the wagon as some people find themselves craving simple carbs again after one pass.

If you find yourself facing a social situation where you know that cake, pizza or other carb heavy foods will be present and not much else, there is something that you can do to be able to indulge a little bit. Indulge here means a slice of pizza or cake and not the whole pie, or seconds and thirds. This is the only exception to the rule and should not be an everyday or even every week occurrence, lest it become the rule.

Obviously, when eating out I'd prefer if you went for the salad or fruit or any other natural whole foods that hasn't gone through much processing, but knowing human nature I am aware a calculated cheat is ten times better than a non-calculated cheat, so I'll provide you with a way to make the most of the situation many of you will find yourselves in.

The only time when consuming a simple carb will not hinder your fat loss progress so much, will be after a hard and heavy weight training work out session. A lot of your glycogen stores in the muscle are depleted when you do a heavy resistance/weight training work out session, so when you consume sugars/carbs after such a session, your food will actually go towards repairing the muscle tissue instead of being converted directly to fat.

What happens is your insulin level will spike to shuttle carbs/sugars in the blood to the muscles that you have just worked. Keep in mind though that once the muscles are filled, any excess will be stored as fat. Unfortunately, these foods tend to be much more calorie dense, hence why this hack is being recommended as a once in a blue moon technique for when you want to join in on the holiday/work festivities.

The key to applying this hack the right way is to make sure that you do not resistance train the legs heavily, but rather the upper body because this technique is commonly used for muscle building purposes (see carb cycling vs. calorie cycling). This doesn't mean you need 1000 lb dumbbells, 5 pounds are fine; just make sure you are training the upper body with weights to failure.

You also need to be cognizant of the amount of calories you have left in your day/eating window and whatever you do, don't exceed your TDEE as shown by your HRM or the numbers provided by an online calculator with a sedentary activity level plus your individual workout calories burned for the day. Finally, if you do eat again try to follow the Hunger Training Protocol™ to wait until all the food from your cheat has been used up for energy.

HIGH FIBER

High-fiber diets are excellent for those seeking to lose fat. Not only does it help ward off many diseases, it has been shown to aid in weight loss by reducing food intake at meals. Fiber in general is good for digestive health as it is a substance that our body cannot break down and absorb and therefore helps keep our bowel movements regular.

There are two types of fiber, soluble and insoluble fiber, neither of which can be absorbed by the body. They have different properties when mixed with water, hence the designation between the two. Soluble fiber binds a small amount of protein and fat in the stomach carrying it out without digestion. So if you amp up soluble fiber intake, you end up absorbing less of the calories that go into your mouth as much of it will be lost in the bathroom. Insoluble fiber does not absorb or dissolve in water. It passes through our digestive system in close to its original form.

When determining the carbohydrate content of a food, you should subtract the amount of fiber from the overall carbohydrates to determine the net carbs. For example, if a food has 25 grams of carbs and 10 grams of that is fiber, you only count 15 net carbs, because that's all the body will be absorbing for energy.

In terms of where you'll get the most dietary fiber, it is found only in plant products. Thus, nuts, legumes, fruits and vegetables, will be your best source of fiber. I would caution you to stay away from fiber supplements and get it from whole foods instead, because supplements don't provide the vitamins, minerals and other nutrients that fiber-rich foods do, may reduce blood sugar levels and could reduce or delay how your body absorbs other nutrients from food.

LOW SUGAR (NO ADDED SUGAR)

Different foods affect the body in different ways and sugar is uniquely fattening. First, let me clarify what sugar is so that we are all on the same page.

Sugar is the generalized name for a class of chemically-related sweet-flavored substances, most of which are used as food. They are carbohydrates, composed of carbon, hydrogen and oxygen. As you are well aware at this point in the book, I am not a big fan of simple carbohydrates, which the bodies views as sugar, but it's not without good reason. Re-read the low-carb section if you need a quick reminder.

There are various types of sugar derived from different sources. Simple sugars are called monosaccharides and include glucose (also known as dextrose), fructose and galactose. Most people hear sugar and think of basic table sugar, the white crystals used in most homes and in much cooking. This sugar is called sucrose and comes from sugar beets or sugarcane. Sucrose is a disaccharide (in the body, sucrose hydrolyses into fructose and glucose) and is broken down to glucose and fructose almost immediately. Other disaccharides include maltose and lactose.

Chemically-different substances may also have a sweet taste, but are not classified as sugars. Some are used as lower-calorie food substitutes for sugar described as artificial sweeteners.11

It is important to note here that the body doesn't always know the difference and artificial sweeteners have been shown to generate an insulin response similar to sugar.

There are very little redeeming qualities to sugar. Amongst the list of destruction sugar boasts, it promotes fat storage and weight gain, decreases your body's production of leptin (the hormone critical for appetite regulation), spurs insulin resistance, and is pro-aging due to oxidative stress on the body. On top of all this, high doses of sugar trigger the same endorphin response as hard drugs.

It is incredibly difficult to remove sugar from your diet 100%, as it is found in fruits and other whole foods. However, when preparing your own meals from home it is entirely possible to abstain from adding sugar (white, brown or otherwise) to your meals. If absolutely necessary opt for raw honey or coconut sugar, but be aware that cooking or heating kills the good stuff in honey.

---

[11] Wikipedia - en.wikipedia.org/wiki/Sugar

The best way to become accustomed to the taste of food without sugar is to stop feeding the sugar taste buds cold turkey. It's up to you how strictly you want to adhere to sugars that naturally appear in more nutritious foods, like fruits, but I would advise you to pay attention to the overall sugar content before nutritional benefits and treat fruit with higher sugar content as a garnish or treat. As for a numerical number for exactly how much sugar to take in, lump it under carbs, which should be kept around 50g, and no more than 100g per day.

LOW SODIUM

You know that water weight low carb dieters are accused of losing over fat? It's very real; but weight gain in the form of water retention/water weight has another culprit and salt, which is made up of sodium, is its name. Sodium triggers one's thirst mechanism as it reduces the concentration of electrolytes in the blood. To balance the electrolyte concentration in your body, kidneys retain water. This increases the water concentration in the blood; it moves to different body tissues, making them swell.

While our daily sodium needs ranges from 180-500 mg and the recommended level is set at 1,500, currently the average sodium intake from ages 2 and up is 3,400 mg.[12] The worst offenders contributing to the sky-high salt intake are foods prepared at restaurants and sold as over-processed grocery products as may items marketed as low in calories, make up for it in carbs and sodium. After all, how else could they stay fresh without artificial ingredients, and salt?

Filling an empty stomach with salt will have the same effect on your appetite as overdosing in sugar or caffeine. Too much salt increases an appetite for more salt, which will inevitably be accompanied by trans fats or processed flour. It's an endless cycle that will undoubtedly lead to overeating and bloating. Furthermore, evidence from studies suggests that excess dietary salt and caloric intake, common in diets rich in processed foods, is linked not only to increased blood pressure,

---

[12] U.S. Department of Health and Human Services, U.S. Department of Agriculture. Dietary guidelines for Americans 2010. Washington, DC: Government Publishing Office, 2010.

but also to defective insulin sensitivity, blood glucose levels and thereby obesity.

For those of you addicted to salt, throw out the processed foods, use sea salts for a more flavorful seasoning in cooking and baking, replace salted nuts with raw nuts and try adding your favorite herbs and spices in substitute of salt.

MODERATE FAT

Dietary fat is the only one of the three macronutrients that does not cause insulin release. Therefore, foods made up entirely or predominantly of fat is the only type of food that does not cause any or a significant amount of insulin release. Note that this categorization does not apply to type I diabetics, who are not able to produce insulin at all.

By no means should you pig out on high fat foods all day in hopes of losing weight though. Calories still count and you'll notice, the diet recommendation is for moderate fat. You are still to watch your fat intake and not go overboard.

It may seem pretty obvious, but when you lower one macronutrient, you tend to replace it with another. In this instance, we're doing that with carbs and fat. A primary benefit for relying on fat for calories over predominately relying on carbs is that eating more fat leads to great satiety and fullness over time, and hence, you aren't eating as many calories. Fat in diet also allows the body to absorb vitamins.

MODERATE TO HIGH PROTEIN

Eating moderate to high protein is important for fat/weight loss because it helps preserve lean muscle, which is important in keeping a higher metabolism. Those who do not agree with moderate to high protein diets argue that protein causes an insulin spike just like carbs and thus eating too much of it will cause the body to turn it into sugar, thus making the moderate to high protein suggestion over high carbs, null.

While it is true that protein will release some insulin (although much less than carbs), protein results in the release of glucagon, a hormone that does much of the opposite of insulin.

On top of this, some proteins are more easily assimilated/digested than others. Finally, protein has been shown to have the most effect on satiation. Think about how easy it is to overeat on chips vs. steak.

HACK TIP

COOKING MEAT

By the way, keep in mind a "greasy" burger, whether we're talking beef, chicken, or any other meat, cooked on an actual wire grill will always be better than one cooked on a flat top since fat cooks off, instead of being cooked in. Make a makeshift grill by spraying a little non-stick spray on your oven rack and putting your meat right on it, as well as placing a pan right below the meat to catch any drippings. Alternatively, racks from toaster ovens placed atop a shallow baking pan or pot would work as well.

HIGH NUTRITION / WHOLE FOODS

Whole foods are foods that are unprocessed and unrefined, or processed and refined as little as possible, before being consumed. It's not just vegetables and fruits, but choosing a skinless chicken breast over processed chicken nuggets is one example of a whole food and its highly processed counterpart. Whole foods offer better nutrition than processed foods because during manufacturing many healthy nutrients are removed. For example, whole foods are loaded with vitamins, minerals, fibers and phytochemicals (the natural compounds in plants that protect cells against damage).

Sometimes, nutrients are artificially added back into foods lost in the manufacturing process, but the final product is likely to be less nutritious than the original. Furthermore, the other stuff that gets added, like salt, sugar, preservatives and chemicals, can be a huge problem with processed foods. The extras can lead to calories quickly adding up.

High-nutrition foods are those we know to be really good for us: organic meat, eggs, fish, nonfat and low-fat dairy foods, and lots of fruits and vegetables. These are the foods that are primarily on the perimeter of the grocery aisles. They are also available everywhere and much cheaper than processed foods, since monetary 'value' goes up the more you add to a food (e.g. - apple vs. apple juice).

LOW TO NO DAIRY

Dairy has very specific insulinogenic and appetite increasing properties13. The culprits partially, or wholly, responsible for the insulinemic response of most dairy are whey protein and casein (proteins found in milk). Specifically, they cause an increased insulin response relative to other proteins, as well as a fairly significant IGF-1 (insulin growth factor hormone) response, which causes all tissues to grow. Besides being high fat and calorie dense, each bite of hard cheese has ten times whatever is in a sip of milk (IGF-1) since it takes ten pounds of milk to make one pound of cheese, each bite of ice cream has 12 times, and every swipe of butter 21 times whatever is contained in the fat molecules in a sip of milk. That would all be well and good if you were trying to get bigger and fatter, but I highly suspect you aren't.

[13] Effect of increased dairy consumption on appetitive ratings and food intake, Obesity (Silver Spring). 2007 Jun;15(6):1520-6.

Whey protein is also one of the fastest absorbing proteins available and is fully digested by your body within an hour. Thus, body builders and those trying to get bigger muscles suggest its use in acute states of muscle catabolism, e.g. after a workout or upon waking in the morning. That means if you drink whey in the morning, as most people consume milk with their candy (cereal), not only will your insulin spike and turn off your fat-burning switch, you'll be hungry again within an hour. Just in case I haven't made my position clear, all of the above is a complete recipe for disaster when it comes to contouring a thigh gap.

Now, I understand some of you may love dairy, and although it's truly not helping your cause, want to know if there are any exceptions at all to my no/low dairy rule. There is a way for you to get your milk fix by turning to coconut milk or almond milk, with coconut milk being the lower calorie and tastier (in my opinion) option.

As for cheese, sparingly using goat or sheep cheese, which are low lactose, are going to be better than other types of cheese and fat-free imitation cheese. Remember, we want whole, natural foods and not food made in a science lab out of substances our bodies are not physically able to process. In the case of fat-free cheese, gums and stabilizers are used to simulate the creamy texture and rich taste of regular cheese. I recommend goat or sheep cheese because the casein is usually much better tolerated than cow's casein as goats have been domesticated for much longer than cows have. It is higher in nutrients, lower in fat and digests much easier in our systems. Still, sparingly is the operative word. In other words, don't go overboard and pile goat cheese on to every meal.

MIRACLE FOOD HACKS

Having the basic guidelines to your diet is all well and good, but I find that individual foods and tricks for easy and foolproof implementation are greatly appreciated. I love to cook and despite mastering the basics of what I eat, I absolutely love finding out new low calorie dense foods that fill me up and never have me feeling deprived. In my opinion, the foods I am about to disclose below are miracle foods, but they only barely scratch the surface of delicious foods you can enjoy while keeping your weight in check.

I urge you to go out as soon as you can and make the items that you like staples in your diet! For those of you who may want more in depth guidance in terms of shopping lists and recipes, those details can be found at www.thefemininecontour.com, where you can also sign up for custom weekly meal plans.

NEGATIVE CALORIE FOODS

The thought of negative (or zero) calorie foods is intriguing, since we are used to associating food with supplying energy, in many cases too much energy (hence why we get fat). For the sake of clarity, negative calorie foods supposedly take more energy to digest than they provide in calories. These foods only have this negative calorie effect when consumed without extras added to them like butter, sugar or dips.

While there is no scientific evidence that digestion will require as many calories as the food you are eating is true, it is theoretically possible that this phenomenon can exist. Even if the negative calorie aspect wasn't quite right, and you were to eat a close to zero calorie food, eating low calorie foods in place of high calorie foods will fill you up and typically provide nutritional content your body needs. For example, the poster child of the negative calorie food is celery. Should you eat celery with one tablespoon of peanut butter, you would feel fuller than eating a tablespoon of peanut butter alone and thus more satisfied/full. Without the celery stick, you might have been compelled to have two tablespoons of peanut butter. Since the celery is so low calorie, while you would still need to count the peanut butter (and celery calories) you would reap the benefit of feeling fuller and eating less.

It should be noted that the only truly negative calorie beverage is ice water, which has no calories, but requires the body to expend some energy to raise the liquid to body temperature.

MIRACLE HACKS FOR SUGAR LOVERS

As you know, sugar is addictive and I encourage you to go cold turkey since artificial sweeteners are just as bad as the real thing. However, if you insist on putting up a fight, I want to tell you a true miracle hack that can give you a little bit of the best of both worlds: a kick of sweetness without the Calories and huge insulin spikes.

MIRACLE FRUIT BERRIES

Synsepalum Dulcificum, also known as the miracle fruit berries, originates from West Africa and is a plant with a berry that, when eaten, causes sour foods (such as lemons and limes) subsequently consumed to taste sweet. This effect is due to miraculin, which is used commercially as a sugar substitute.

The berry itself is tasteless and has a low sugar content, which means no crazy insulin spike, but when the fleshy part of the fruit is sucked, chewed or eaten, this molecule binds to the tongue's taste buds, causing bitter and sour foods to taste sweet without a trace of sourness until the protein is washed away by saliva (up to about 60 minutes). Some report the miraculin loses its potency sooner if you use it with a drink than if you use it with food, as the potency goes away as fast as much you are "washing" your mouth.

This fruit is natural, and totally safe with no side effects, so if you want a hack to help you give up the sugar, while still satisfying your taste for it every now and then, invest in these berries. When I say invest, I mean it; It can be a costly experience with one berry costing $2.50. According to the New York Times, 30 of them shipped overnight from Florida will run you $90.

They are also very perishable, quickly turning brown and unappealing. Therefore, you might want to purchase a plant to grow your own if you live in a warm climate like Florida, or consider purchasing the tablets instead. Thinkgeek.com and Miracletaste.com are reputable sources for the tablets, but a quick search on the Internet will provide you with other suppliers.

To use them, simply chew the berries before your meal. You can also take them before having water with lime/lemon for a juice style drink or unsweetened tea with lime/lemon since you should not be drinking your Calories otherwise. Some already low calorie items to try the miracle berries with include tomatoes, 100% plain yogurt, and rhubarb. Pour some lime over your salad for a sweet and low calorie salad dressing or chop up a granny smith apple with Brussels sprouts.

For dessert-like treats, you might also try coconut or almond flour pancakes with lemon, lime and or grapefruit juice in the batter to forgo honey and syrup, or coconut or almond flour cupcakes with goat cheese, cottage cheese or cream cheese spreading to replace the frosting. For warmer months, combine lime juice, crushed mint and water for a lime mojito or crushed ice and strawberries or blueberries with ground flaxseed for filling sugar free smoothies.

My final caution is to use this hack sparingly, not only to save your wallet, but again because chasing the sugar dragon, even if it's technically nutritionally viable, may result in only keeping your cravings going strong.

HACK TIP

NATURAL SUGAR SUBSTITUTES

Substitute fruits for added sugars in your diet. Instead of adding sugar, honey or other sweeteners to cereal and oatmeal, for example, top your serving with fresh-cut apples, bananas or peaches. Fructose is metabolized almost exclusively in the liver (quite in fact almost zero incoming fructose will ever reach the bloodstream in humans) and this is a rate-limited process.

Above a certain point, fructose starts being converted to fat in the liver.14

A tip for those of you used to drinking sweetened juice is to replace them with Celestial herbal tea, the kind with the blueberry, cherry, raspberry and orange lackets included. You won't need sugar with these teas as they is naturally sweet.

Another way to get a sweet taste without adding sugar is to caramelize foods through sautéing or roasting. For example, roasting or sautéing butternut squash, sweet potatoes, bell peppers, garlic and onions until browned will bring out the natural sweetness in them. This should help satisfy your taste for sugar without having to turn to sugar filled "junk foods" like candy bars.

MIRACLE HACKS FOR CARB LOVERS

14 Body Recomposition - www.bodyrecomposition.com/research-review/the-effect-of-two-energy-restricted-diets-a-low-fructose-diet-vs-a-moderate-natural-fructose-diet-research-review.html

SHIRATAKI NOODLES

You love your pasta and one of the biggest gripes you have with The Thigh Gap Diet™ is that in order to meet your fat loss needs you are going to need to ditch starchy, high carb foods. Sure, there are some pasta brands out there that are selling you on how you can have your pasta and eat it too, like Dreamfields™, which claim their "patent-pending" (since 2004) recipe and manufacturing process protects carbs from being digested. Unfortunately, many report that not being the case, and countless studies and personal testimonies have shown insulin spikes mimicking normal pasta. Thus, I suggest you go a safer route to get your pasta fix.

Sometimes called konnyaku noodles, Shiratake noodles is a zero calorie, zero carb miracle that you've probably never heard of. Glucomannan, a water-soluble dietary fiber made from the roots of the Asian Konjac plant, make up the majority of substance in shirataki noodles. Eating lots of dietary fiber, which is found only in plant foods such as whole grains, fruits, vegetables, beans, seeds and nuts, has been proven to have many health benefits.

In addition to the numerous health benefits, eating lots of fiber-rich foods like Shirataki noodles can help you lose weight as fiber itself has no Calories and is passed through your digestive system intact. However, because fiber absorbs water, it provides a "full" feeling. When you feel full, eating is usually the further thing from your mind and when you are eating less but still satiated that is the perfect recipe for weight and fat loss.

Shirataki noodles are packaged "wet" in liquid, and are ready-to-eat out of the package. They have no taste and will absorb whatever spices and sauces you put on them. You can prepare them by boiling them briefly or running them under hot water, then roasting them in a dry pan for a few minutes before adding things like tofu, garlic, spinach, tomato sauce, or soy sauce to enhance the flavor.

KELP NOODLES

Much like Shirataki noodles, when eating Kelp noodles, calories can be the furthest worry from your mind. At just 6 calories per serving, these noodles are made out of sea kelp, and packed with water. Yet they perform amazingly well in soups, raw noodle dishes and even Italian-style dishes like spaghetti. They take up a lot of physical space in your belly, contributing to that "full" feeling that reminds you to stop eating.

SPAGHETTI SQUASH

Another option for you pasta lovers out there is to discover vegetables that you can prepare as you would pasta, but offer much lower calories and much higher nutritional value, such as spaghetti squash. Spaghetti Squash is low in calories, with an ounce worth of cooked squash only translating to a measly 13 calories and approximately 2 net carbs. One whole medium sized spaghetti squash will set you back around 142 calories and fill you up for hours. Plus, the strands look amazingly similar to actual spaghetti, especially when covered in tomato sauce, which does have an effect making you feel as though you are indulging in the real thing.

The best way to prepare spaghetti squash is to cut it in half and scoop out the seeds and innards before placing it face side down in a bowl with a ¼ to ½ a cup of water. Next, put the bowl in a 400-degree oven for one hour. Remove and let cool before turning the squash face side up and scooping out the squash with a fork or spoon. I like to then sauté it garlic, basil, peppers, onions and one serving of tomato sauce low in sugar and carbs. Depending on how you cook the squash, there may be a sweet taste to the strands that will have you returning to this dish often.

ZUCCHINI SQUASH

One of my all time favorite pasta alternatives is Zucchini Squash. At only 5 Calories per ounce, this low calorie and low carb summer squash makes for an amazing dish when shredded and cooked in light pasta sauce. All it takes is running a vegetable peeler on the green outer skin of the squash to reveal the flesh, then using the same peeler, mandolin or spiralizer to make long strips of zucchini ribbons that resemble fettuccine pasta. You want to strip the squash until you come across the seeds and then stop. Cook the strands of "noodles" by quickly sautéing them with a little olive oil, garlic, peppers and/or herbs and spices. Then, add one serving of low sugar/carb/calorie tomato sauce or pesto and enjoy!

BREAD SUBSTITUTES

Surely, you've heard about whole wheat bread being better for you than white bread, but when put to the test, the glycemic index of whole wheat ranges between 68 and 85, (high) just like that of white bread. The truth of the matter is the effect on insulin levels from eating whole wheat bread isn't any different than with white bread, so if you can, avoid both.

I realize saying cut out bread to someone who lives for endless breadbaskets and garlic knots, examples of two of my personal previous weaknesses, seems darn near impossible. However, when you think about it, bread simply provides a shuttle for protein and fat, you know – the real food you enjoy. It also adds volume to your meal (makes you feel fuller). You can replicate the effects of bread by getting a little creative with other foods so that they do the same thing bread does, only for fewer calories and less insulin spike.

My go-to bread substitutes are roasted or grilled eggplants sliced in the shape of discs, roasted bell peppers sliced lengthwise, Portobello mushrooms with the gills cut out and Chinese cabbage for tortilla rolls.

HACKS FOR SNACKS

Generally, when you develop and adjust to the Thigh Gap Diet™, you will find your cravings for snacks drastically diminish because you'll be getting nutritious and filling foods that should hold you over between meals.

Snacks are synonymous with high carb diets because once a high insulin spike gets to work on removing all of the toxic sugars out of your blood, you are left with an unbalanced blood sugar level, which leaves you hungry very soon after eating. Although I'd much rather prefer you prepare a full meal I understand every now and then you might just want a quick snack and so here are some of the best options for when those times occur.

Ideally, your snacks should be in accordance with the guidelines I have given you above. It should be a whole food, have moderate/high protein, fat and fiber, and low carbohydrates, sugar and salt. Since your goal with snacking is fulfilling hunger between meals and we know that protein trumps carbohydrates and fat for blunting hunger, protein is the most important element of your snack.

KALE

The secret about Kale is out. Every time I go to my grocery store later than 9am the kale section is guaranteed to be bare, and there is a good reason. Kale is low in calories and packed in nutrients. It also tastes delicious and is super simple to cook. The latest snack craze is kale chips. These goodies sell for around $7 to $8 per bag, but are very easy to make yourself. Separate kale from the stems, drizzle with a little bit of extra virgin olive oil and a pinch of salt (although not necessary) and your favorite herbs/spices before baking in the oven for 15 or so minutes or until the leaves are formed to your desired crispiness.

MULTI-COLORED BELL PEPPERS

Have you discovered the yummy goodness, bell peppers? Roasted bell peppers and quick and easy to cook and taste delicious by itself or as a shuttle for protein as opposed to bread. You can slice a bell pepper in half and crack an egg white inside it before baking it, or simply eat it with a piece of lean meat. You can also eat the peppers raw with hummus.

ORGANIC POPCORN

Popcorn is a whole grain food that is not only low in calories, but also a good source of fiber. This means it takes longer to chew and makes you feel full longer. Compared to many snack foods, popcorn is low in calories. One whole cup of popcorn is a serving, with air-popped popcorn providing only 30 calories per cup and oil-popped containing only 55 calories.

However, popcorn does contain a good amount of carbohydrates and most people can only tolerate 15 grams of net carbs per meal, therefore I recommend consuming no more than 3 cups of popped popcorn at a time otherwise blood sugars will start to go up. Also, be sure to check the ingredients in popcorn and steer clear of popcorn that is not organic, as it could be genetically modified, mixed with vegetable oil that isn't organic and any salt other than sea salt (if you pop your own popcorn don't bother adding the salt or butter).

RAW NUTS

We've already covered salted nuts not being so good for you, but raw nuts are great by themselves as a snack or in a salad. There are too many kinds to count, but some of the better-known and more popular ones include almonds, cashews, hazel nuts, Brazil nuts, walnuts and peanuts. Interestingly, some are fruits in and of themselves, and others are the seeds of other fruits. We call them all nuts. While nuts are reasonable choices for a whole food snack, they are very high in calories and easy to overeat, therefore they must be weighed and limited to one ounce per serving.

SWEET POTATOES

Finally, one of my meal staples that can also be eaten as a snack is roasted sweet potato. Sweet potatoes baked in the skin without salt equals 26 calories per ounce. This is how I prefer to eat my sweet potatoes, but the 45-minute to one-hour cooking time may not meet the requirements of a quick snack, although you could always prepare them in advance and reheat in the oven.

If you are running short on time there is a way to enjoy sweet potatoes as a snack. Just peel one sweet potato, cut into wedges (the smaller and thinner the wedge, the faster the cooking time) and drizzle with a bit of extra virgin olive oil. Chop up liberal amounts of garlic and add to the baking dish along with cinnamon (you'll see why in a minute) and your favorite herbs and spices. Bake or roast for 20 to 30 minutes, let cool and eat up.

HACK TIPS

COOKING OIL

One of the glaring omissions I see in clients' food diaries is that of cooking oil. I'm pretty sure most people are not steaming their meals and in fact drenching them in tasty oils, so leaving this essential fat, which holds 9 Calories per gram (by far the most of the macronutrients), out of their food logs is in my opinion, sacrilegious.

Before I included cooking oils the Calories of my meals were 50% underestimated! That's because one tablespoon of olive oil is 120 Calories. So, my 150-calorie meal was actually more like 300 Calories! And we have already covered the danger in working with wrong numbers. That is why I am going to caution you to learn to measure your cooking oil before including it in your meal! None of this whirling the bottle wildly into your pan as though you were one of the chefs on The Food Network.

Some helpful shortcuts include measuring how much one capful of olive oil is one time and forever knowing how many capfuls you should use in your meal. For example, one capful of my brand of olive oil measures out to be 5 grams. Since one teaspoon (120 Calories) is approximately 15 grams, I know I can add up to 3 capfuls of oil per meal, however I shoot for more like one.

Another way to hack the oil calorie fest is to place foods in a zip lock bag, add seasoning and a measured amount of olive oil before shaking vigorously. This evenly distributes the amount of oil all of your food and works particularly well for grilled vegetables.

Finally, you can turn to cooking sprays, but note cooking sprays in an aerosol can include propellants which is why I recommend looking into The Misto. The Misto works with air pressure so there is nothing but organic oil going on your food (or whatever type of oil you choose to fill it with). It sprays just like an aerosol, you just have to pump the lid every once in awhile to build up the pressure. The Misto can be found in my store, at www.thighgaphack.com/products

METABOLISM BOOSTING SPICES

GARLIC – When it comes to weight loss, garlic is a miracle food. It contains the compound allicin, which has anti-bacterial effects and helps reduce unhealthy fats and cholesterol. It also boosts your metabolism, eliminates fat from the cell, is an effective diuretic and regulates sharp ups and downs in your blood sugar levels that cause carbs and sweets cravings and fat storing.

Raw garlic needs to interact with oxygen to form allicin, the active ingredient that helps the most with your health. 15 Therefore, to make sure you reap all the health benefits of garlic, crush it and let it sit in the open air 10 minutes before using it. Generally, the stronger the taste, the higher the health benefits of garlic. It should also be noted that allicin is destroyed in cooking, but other helpful compounds are formed, so cooked garlic is still healthy. However, you can pass on processed garlic powder or garlic salt, as most of the healthy ingredients are long gone by then.

CINNAMON - In a recent article in the Journal of Agricultural and Food Chemistry, chemist Richard A. Anderson co-authored a study with colleagues at the Beltsville (Maryland) Human Nutrition Research Center and two universities. In test tubes containing fat cells, the "polyphenolic polymers"

---

[15] www.brainyweightloss.com/health-benefits-of-garlic.html

associated with cinnamon bark were found to increase sugar metabolism a whopping 20-fold.16 How so?

An Insulin Mimicker creates the artificial appearance of insulin to your body, still escorting the sugar you ingest into the appropriate areas of your body, but without the harmful spike that can lead to fat storage, insulin resistance, and even possibly Type 2 Diabetes17.

Sprinkle cinnamon over fruit or savory items such as baked sweet potato or mushrooms and of course you can add it to your green tea each morning in place of a cup of coffee to get the antioxidants you need to remain healthy and keep that insulin in check!

─────────────────────

[16] (Source: United States Department of Agriculture Agricultural Research Service)

[17] United States Department of Agriculture Agricultural Research Service

A word of Caution - Don't take cinnamon first thing in the morning as your blood sugar is already low upon waking and you don't want to risk a hypoglycemic reaction, causing you to pass out during a morning workout.

SUCCESSFUL DIET ADHERANCE

Following the diet I've laid out for you and using some of the specific food hacks above serves two primary functions: to help you reach satiation, and keep you sated longer when you eat your meals. To achieve satiation filling up the stomach, along with some other factors, will do the trick, whereas satiety is achieved by providing the body with quality nutrients and fuel that burns slow and steady for a longer time.

Generally, it is much easier to be satiated than sated since it takes about 3 hours for the nutrients to reach the small intestine that tell us we do not need any more food. Thus, while it is good to focus on getting the most nutrient and energy dense food, a true hacker would try to manipulate satiation. As it turns out, I've already put a lot of thought and research into that very thing.

DON'T HIDE FATS

One hack proven to manipulate satiation is making fat visible as opposed to hiding them in your meals. In the study, Hidden Fat Facilitates Passive Overconsumption, it was concluded that in the presence of visible fats, energy intake was lower than in the presence of hidden fats, suggesting that hidden fats may contribute to overconsumption. The effect was 8-9%, minor but significant.18 It goes to show our perceptions do not perfectly estimate the nutritive content of foods.

EAT SLOWER AND TAKE SMALLER BITES

Another study showed that satiation is also affected by how fast we eat and how big of a bite we take. In this study, not

---

[18] Mirre Viskaal-van Dongen, Cees de Graaf, Els Siebelink, and Frans J. Kok. Hidden Fat Facilitates Passive Overconsumption. J. Nutr. February 2009 vol. 139 no. 2 394-399

eating slowly and taking small bites led to people eating up to 50% more than when they were limited to small bites every nine seconds. Thus, the researchers concluded "Greater oral sensory exposure to a product, by eating with small bite sizes rather than with large bite sizes and increasing OPT [oral processing time], significantly decreases food intake."19

EAT SMALLER MEALS

One of the huge benefits to eating smaller meals is that over time, doing so will decrease the stomach. What does this mean? A human stomach is extremely flexible. It can shrink and stretch very easily. Our stomachs shrinks less and more slowly than it can stretch however. When you eat larger meals the stomach stretches more. In fact, some gastric bypass patients have over-eaten to the point of re-stretching their surgically altered stomachs back to their (nearly) normal size.

---

[19] Nicolien Zijlstra, René de Wijk, Monica Mars, Annette Stafleu, and Cees de Graaf. Effect of bite size and oral processing time of a semisolid food on satiation. Am J Clin Nutr August 2009 vol. 90 no. 2 269-275

As you can imagine, a tummy that is smaller will signal that you are full faster than a tummy that is larger.

VOLUME EATING

The capacity a stomach can hold is based on volume, and as we've already covered, how much the stomach has been stretched. It has been purported the average human stomach can hold 2 to 4 liters of food20 or up to 2.5 lbs of food, water or both. It's worth noting that if you were to eat very dense foods or liquids, you could very well hold more than 2.5 pounds of food in your stomach.

Slightly related to eating smaller meals, not eating more than a certain volume of food in one sitting is a precise way to control food intake, especially since volume partially determines when we feel full, and help shrink the stomach. For example, I could say aim for 300 to 400 calorie meals but that could go very far

[20] Curtis, Helena & N. Sue Barnes. *Invitation to Biology*. 5th Edition. New York: Worth, 1994: 529.

or very little depending on the food. While dividing up calories across the amount of times you choose to eat per day (I recommend 3) is a great idea, eating by volume is an excellent trick one can use to assist with diet adherence.

Basically, the gist of this method is to eat no more than 1 pound of food at a sitting/meal (naturally you can elect to stop eating before reaching that number) and to drink at least one cup of water 10 or so minutes before consuming your meal. One pound equates to 16 ounces of food and one cup of water equates to 8 ounces of liquid, for a total of 1.5 pounds.

No, this does not mean you can eat whatever you want as long as it is less than 16 ounces. If you implement this rule for yourself and apply them to the whole foods I covered in the chapters above you will be fine, especially since whole foods are more nutrient dense than processed foods. Of course, it is important to remember that overcall calories matter – but using this self-imposed rule can help keep you in check so that you do not overeat, even on the good stuff.

DON'T DRINK AND EAT

When you drink while eating, especially carbonated beverages such as seltzer water, it forces food through the stomach pouch faster. That means food does not stay in your pouch as long and you lose the feeling of satiety and increase the chances that you will eat more. Finally, the gas released from the carbonated beverage may cause the food forced through the pouch to enlarge your stoma, which again would allow you to eat more at one sitting.

This is why I do not recommend eating and drinking at the same time, or even drinking anything besides water and tea (you should not be drinking away your precious calories). By all means, drink as much ice cold water (see cold therapy) as you want throughout the day and a few minutes before meals to help you eat less overall, but not while eating.

3 FOODS/INGREDIENTS RULE

When I visited China a few years ago, every restaurant served up huge meals on Lazy Susans. The selections ran the gamut of meats, vegetables, sides, etc. When faced with all of these options I found myself trying a little bit of this and a little bit of that. You may relate if you've ever gotten food from food buffets and cafeterias or all you can eat restaurants.

The only reason I probably didn't balloon up on my trip was because of all the exercising/walking we were doing as tourists and the lack of sweets in Chinese meals. The standard dessert was sliced oranges as opposed to chocolate mousse or cake (typical desserts of choice for Americans include a lot of fat, carbs and sugar). Since most of you reading this in fact spend the majority of your days doing the exact opposite (sitting in front of a computer) I do not recommend this way of eating.

It's human nature to eat whatever food is presented before us and end up overeating until our plates are clean. Thus, limiting the amount of foods on your plate to no more than three foods is an effective hack against overeating.

What do I mean by no more than three foods? When fixing yourself a plate of food, include one lean meat or protein, one low carb starch, such as sweet potatoes or vegetables (a salad would count as one item, and a variety of grilled vegetables such as red and green peppers would count as one item), and a small amount of fat (e.g. – hummus, goat cheese, oil over vinegar) is one manner of composing your meals according to this hack. You could also elect to have less than 3 items if you so desire.

MEAL PLANNING

There are two approaches you can take when it comes to meal planning: calculate as you go or prepare in advance. Hacking your way to thin thighs will mean that you need to be precise and use the best method to bring about our results in the quickest amount of time.

Most people take a calculate as you go approach which entails not pre planning your meals or ingredients and adding your Calories up throughout the day as you go along, while trying to stay within your caloric limit for the day. So, for example, a woman who has 1500 Calories to work with in the day might awake and decide to make breakfast. She would then get her ingredients out, weight them, and either write them down manually or using a convenient calorie-tracking program such as myfitnesspal.com or fitday.com

She would then discover that her meal has cost her 500 Calories and she is left with 1000 for the day. Then, the same woman goes to work and buys a sandwich containing 400 Calories. That brings her down to 600 Calories left for the day. She may then grab a drink from the store that costs her 300 Calories. 300 left. As she is home trying to prepare dinner and fit it into 400 Calories she may find herself struggling to do so.

Do you want to know a better approach? Why, of course you do!

HOW TO DO IT

Pre-constructing your meals simply means planning what you are going to eat based on your allotted Calories and sticking to it, but instead of coming up with what you are going to eat on the fly and then trying to calculate your Calories, you will have a few staple meals that you will easily be able to create and know for sure how many Calories you are consuming.

The benefits include not having to think about what you are going to eat every second of the day and not having to log Calories or look up Calories for specific foods for every single meal. Remember, the easier you can make this process the more likely you will stick to it and get the desired results.

The trick is to keep on target with recipes and not deviate, as this will alter the amount of Calories you are actually consuming. Unsurprisingly, typically those alterations will translate to a higher consumption of Calories.

The easiest way to accomplish this is to search for whole meal recipes according to the amount of Calories in the meal on the Internet. Look out for my new book coming out which will feature 200, 300, and 400-calorie meals. In the meantime, dedicate one day to figuring out the foods you would like to eat and then doing a bit of research online for recipes that include caloric breakdowns or figuring out the Calories yourself. Bookmark these recipes in folders under 200, 300 or 400 calorie labels for easy access. I would recommend you try to include 3 or 4 recipes for light, medium and heavy meals. Once you are finished you will have made make your own personalized recipe book where you store all of your detailed recipes and their nutritional values.

Now, you can flip through your book, browser or through your excel/word documents and pick and choose what to eat without the daily task of calorie counting and looking up or logging nutritional values on my fitness pal or any other similar website.

This may seem very detailed, however taking the time to plot everything out over the course of a day will free up so much of your time in the long run and take away the tedium of having to do this every day. Knowing you have 1200 Calories to consume for the day and being able to easily select two 400 calorie recipes and one 300 calorie meal for the day will save you a lot of time and worry as well as get you to stop obsessing over what you are going to eat next. Also, if you were to go ahead and pre plan your meals for the week, grocery shopping would be a breeze that wouldn't involve impulse buys.

If you're reading this and thinking the monotony of pre-planned meals sounds dreadful, just realize that most of us eat the same meals day in and day out anyway. There really is very little variety to our diets and so having 15 or so pre-planned meals is actually more than enough variety to keep you from getting bored. Plus, these will be meals and foods that you enjoy so you won't get tired. Finally, you will always have the option of adding new recipes to your arsenal at any point in time with a quick search engine inquiry.

HACK TIPS

ROUND UP

A notorious reason people gain weight is that they underestimate how many Calories they are truly consuming from their foods. A great tip for accounting for this is to round up to an even number in increments of 50 when creating your recipes.

MEAL FOR TWO

Since most people work during the day and are unable to prepare a full meal every time they eat (particularly during lunch), one should make their first meal large enough to accommodate 2 separate meals. Yes, that means you will be eating the same thing twice, but that shouldn't matter.

http://www.thighgaphack.com

To help avoid the urge you may get to eat the second meal in the first sitting, pack up the designated proportions in a container, seal it and put it in the fridge to get cold or somewhere out of sight that will require effort to get to.

Part 6 – Exercise Hacks

EXERCISE OVERVIEW

Physical activity reduces weight by increasing the brain's sensitivity to appetite-suppressing hormones like leptin and insulin more so than by burning calories. However, any old exercise will not do when it comes to diminishing stubborn body fat in the hips and thighs to reveal a thigh gap. For our purpose, what you don't do is just as important as what you actually do if you want to avoid bulky legs that are not conducive to the thigh gap.

While we're on the subject, this is the perfect opportunity to address the term 'bulky', since many women are wary of the bulk but told it is as mythical as the Easter Bunny. Bulk is an objective word that varies according to each woman. Women can indeed get bulky, as defined as more muscles than one would like, without taking steroids/drugs and possessing as much testosterone as men. For some reason many 'trainers' and 'experts' like to play dumb as though they cannot fathom the simple concept of a stocky look versus a lithe look. They also play blind and deaf, when you tell them your training sessions are leaving you with larger legs than you'd prefer.

As a gross generalization, women can build lower body muscle at rates comparable to men while men can usually build upper body muscle faster than women. The difference is most men, and some female bodybuilders, say 'bring it on!" to increased leg muscles.

Even the natural female body builders who don't juice, but lift heavy, develop the muscular shoulders, hard lines and overly defined musculature in their quads and hamstrings that plenty of women find undesirable and frankly, too masculine for personal taste. Thus, time and time again, women rebuke muscles, especially for the abs and thighs. The fact is, so many wouldn't echo this concern if it wasn't a real one.

There are a variety of training styles in the fitness arena. Before we get into the specifics of which types of exercise is best for you and why, let's take a look at the main options.

CARDIOVASCULAR/CARDIO

Cardiovascular means heart, thus any exercise that gets your heart rate pumping can be considered cardio. This is anything with relative low intensity that you can do for a prolonged period of time that elevates your heart rate. Regular aerobics, going for a four-mile jog, running on a treadmill for an hour, using the elliptical for twenty minutes, are all examples of cardiovascular exercise. Cardio is considered to be aerobic work.

AEROBICS

Aerobic exercise and cardio exercise are the same thing and although the words stem from different origins, achieve the same results: improved fitness by increasing both your oxygen intake and heart rate. The technic difference between the two is aerobic exercise is defined as exercise that promotes a greater oxygen intake and cardio exercise is exercise that promotes a greater heart rate. Still, you cannot do one without the other, as there is no way you can increase your respiratory rate without also making your heart pump harder and vice versa.

Aerobics is usually performed to music and includes improving flexibility strength and heart and lung fitness, The main components are a warm-up, a conditioning phase using the same large muscle group, rhythmically, where a 60-80% maximum heart rate is maintained for a minimum of 20 to 30 minutes, and a cool-down phase. You should be able to carry on a short conversation while doing aerobic exercise. If you are gasping for air while talking, you are probably not working aerobically, but anaerobically.

INTERVAL TRAINING

Interval training involves alternating sessions of work and recovery and works both anaerobic and aerobic energy systems. When you run, bike, use the elliptical, etc., for periods of speed and intensity followed by periods of rest, you are interval training. An example of an interval training workout would be sprinting for 30 seconds followed by 90 seconds of jogging, and repeating this cycle for 20-30 minutes. This training allows you to work intensely but avoid fatigue as the recovery periods and the level of intensity is related to the length of the work interval. If more effort is required then the work interval is shorter.

There are different levels of interval training one can do. For example, there is high intensity interval training (HIIT), medium intensity interval training and low intensity interval training. At the moment, HIIT is the holy grail of working out, but we will soon examine if there is anything HIIT has to offer those of us working towards a thigh gap. Interval training is considered to be alactic anaerobic work.

CIRCUIT TRAINING

Developed by R.E. Morgan and G.T. Anderson in 1953 at the University of Leeds in England21, circuit training is a form of body conditioning or resistance training using high-intensity aerobics. It targets strength building and muscular endurance by having participants move from one activity to the next after

[21] ^ a b Kraviz, Len (1996-00-00). "New Insights into Circuit Training". University of New Mexico. Retrieved 2006-11-16

completing the required repetitions. This type of training relies heavily on the FITT principle (frequency, intensity, time and type). The aim for each activity is to exercise to overload or failure or near failure and then allow the energy systems to recover to some amount depending on intensity.

An exercise "circuit" is one completion of all prescribed exercises in the program. When one circuit is complete, one begins the first exercise again for the next circuit. Traditionally, the time between exercises in circuit training is short, often with rapid movement to the next exercise.

RESISTANCE / WEIGHT TRAINING

Weight training is a common type of strength training for developing the strength and size of skeletal muscles. It uses the weight force of gravity (in the form of weighted bars, dumbbells, weight stacks or body weight) to oppose the force generated by muscle through concentric or eccentric contraction. Weight training uses a variety of specialized equipment to target specific muscle groups and types of movement and is considered to be anaerobic work.

WHAT TYPE OF WORKOUT TO DO

While 80% of your fat and weight loss will come from the food you ultimately decide to use to fuel your body, exercise plays a role in leaning out your thighs. As I'm sure you already know, your workout can drastically alter your progress. Unfortunately, there is so much misinformation, half-truths, poorly conducted research and flat out myths/lies spread on a daily basis that if you are not careful you can have the exact opposite results of what you are hoping to accomplish.

For example, you may find lots of people touting on message board, especially men, that if you want slim thighs you need to lift a lot of heavy weights while squatting and lunging. Funnily enough, if you search for how to build up the legs/thighs on those very same message boards you'll come across the same advice. You will also find lots of proponents of high intensity interval training programs like Cross Fit and the like, where you train at maximum capacity and then at a much lower capacity, on and off for approximately 15 to 20 minutes total.

The problem is, take one look at the women who train by lifting heavy, going crazy with squats and lunges or doing 15 minute HIIT workouts, and you will quickly realize they do not embody the physique you want. Their thighs are usually thicker than you and I would find ideal or downright muscular, which is okay if that's what they like, but a far cry from the Hollywood, model-like look that we are trying to achieve.

Perhaps now you can understand why I stress the fact that I've put in the work before presenting my findings to you. Only the most credible and proven information has made its way into this book. Let's go through the many misconceptions and frankly, terrible advice given by the "fitness experts" and "fitness message board gurus" and see how it stacks up to the truth below.

There are those who will try to convince you that if you object to wanting to gain mass, something is wrong with you. They assure you that women cannot bulk up without the help of steroids and that lifting heavy weights won't cause you to gain muscle or increased inches on your legs at all.

The truth? When you train a muscle in a certain manner, especially with resistance, it is bound to grow in size and in some instances appear more defined and muscular than you may desire.

The body responds in very specific ways to training. If you do enough training on your legs and "tear" the muscles from fatigue, when it repairs it will do so a little bit stronger and bigger in a calorie surplus, or harder and more defined in a calorie deficit. As you get stronger and progressively add weights, or do more reps in the same period of time it used to take to do a certain set, or exercise longer because you don't feel the same burn as before, you create an environment prime for muscle growth (during a surplus) or retaining lean muscle (during a deficit).

As well, if you aren't getting rid of the layer of fat on top of the muscles through a calorie deficit, (lifting weights solely will not contribute to a deficit as efficiently as cardio) the more developed or newly built muscle will push the fat out, resulting in a wider thigh and making your problem even worst than when you began.

Accompanying the lift heavy mantra is the notion of rep training and the idea that to make the legs smaller, one has to do tons upon tons of reps. This is constantly perpetuated on workout dvds where you're forced to do a million inner thigh leg lifts to "feel the burn", as well as in a plethora of articles targeting women. Unfortunately, or fortunately, it's not true.

First of all, let's define some terms so that we are all on the same page. Low reps are considered to be reps in the 1-5 range taken to failure, as typically used by power lifters for strength training. Mid reps are in the 6-12 range taken to failure, as traditionally used by bodybuilders. Anything above 12 reps taken to failure, we'll call high reps.

Increased muscle size is attributed to sarcoplasmic fluid build-up (the sarcoplasm/cytoplasm of the muscle cells) caused by high volume routines. High rep ranges stimulate muscular endurance, by increasing mitochondrial density within the muscle cell and produces high levels of phosphate and hydrogen ions, which enhance the growth process.

While not being able to stimulate much growth, high reps are very useful for depleting glycogen stores within the muscle.

The body will react to this depletion by increasing muscular glycogen stores. In the long run this will allow cells to stretch and lead to greater overall muscle growth and release of anabolic hormones. It makes sense when you think about it; doing lots of reps will tire your muscles out and they'll start to adapt in ways to prevent them from getting tired as easily.

So, when you embark on a high rep program you will look bigger in the short term because most of the initial size you put on will be intracellular fluid, increased glycogen storage, edema and just overall swelling from the trauma inflicted. You'll also get bigger in the long term.

Does the above mean that you should do low or moderate reps to avoid mass? Not exactly. Moderate rep ranges have consistently been proven to lead to the greatest amount of growth. The reason is that it provides you with the benefits of low rep and high rep training. The heavy loads stimulate myofibrillar hypertrophy (an increase in the number and size of the actin and myosin filaments within muscle tissue), and the increased time under tension stimulates sarcoplasmic hypertrophy.

What of low rep ranges? Low reps are said to contribute to strength gains. However, make the load heavy enough, and do enough sets and guess what? You will see some growth.

If you've been paying attention, you'll notice I've just given you an example of how all three rep ranges can lead to mass and muscle growth. That's because the overarching point is that the body wants to adapt to the stress you are putting it under, which is exactly what lifting heavy is. Progressive overload is the most important principle behind muscle hypertrophy. Progressively increasing intensity, time under load, volume (number of reps, amount of weight, number of sets) and even decreasing rest time between sets is part of progressive overload. Women and men utilizing heavy training target the muscle fibers with the greatest potential for growth and build size and strength more effectively than light training. Thus, if size and strength is not your goal, heavy training shouldn't be your tool of choice. Low volume, low sets and low reps, on the other hand, will be.

Then there is the creative solution to side-stepping the actual problem of wanting thinner thighs, which is to build up your lateral muscles so that your lower body appears smaller. There is nothing I can really say about this because it doesn't even address the problem besides trying to camouflage it. Needless to say, we can safely ignore this unhelpful nugget of wisdom.

The final type of bad advice, which doesn't actually offer a solution but comes from both men and defeated women, is to embrace your strong legs because it's sexy and who would want 'skinny, thin legs' anyway? Well, that's easy – most women. Strong, big, muscular thighs are usually associated with men because that's the build that they want. Train like them and that's exactly what you'll get. Women, on the other hand usually want the complete opposite. It's the whole ying/yang concept. Having said all that, what is the ultimate training regimen for women?

AEROBIC VS. ANAEROBIC

Before the 1990's the general population of the USA embraced aerobic training and running. Then came the 2000's and a revolutionary message had elbowed its way into the spotlight: aerobic work was a time-waster that diminished strength, power and muscle growth.

Arguments against aerobics devolved into comparisons of marathon runners who typically trained for long hours (aerobic or "with oxygen") and sprinters who trained at a high intensity for a short amount of time (anaerobic or "without oxygen"). Since the body is better fueled by oxygen, aerobic training can last for a much longer time than anaerobic training. The sprinters were said to have more "ideal" physiques and thus the aerobic workout videos with the brightly colored leotards became a thing of the past, and hardcore HIIT groups and dvds claimed the throne.

But something should be pointed out here about the "ideal" bodies of the sprinters and the marathon runners. While many sprinters do have very lean and ripped bodies, the body looks thicker, more muscular and you would be hard pressed to find a thigh gap. Meanwhile, the marathon runners are also lean with very lower body fat, but instead of a muscular and thick build, they are slender and thin. You would have a much easier time finding a thigh gap on these women. Thus, for our purposes the "ideal" body is that of the sprinter: lean and lithe.

The reason the two different types of training yield such drastically different body compositions is because of what happens inside the body. When you embark on a high intensity workout, the body will tend to rely more in carbohydrates than oxygen. Anaerobic training is not as sustainable as aerobic, because carbohydrates are stored in the body. When they're gone, they're gone. Oxygen on the other hand is in the air and is extracted with every breath.

To illustrate my point a bit further I am going to get a little deeper and bring talk science with you. There are three types of energy systems that your body uses once you begin to move. The scientific breakdown of each system is as follows[22]:

Alactic Anaerobic: Short term energy; 10 – 15 seconds; ATP-CP Fueled; 1/10th full

Lactic Anaerobic: Mid term energy; 60 – 90 seconds; Glycolysis Fueled; 3/10th full

Aerobic: Long term energy; Hours; Oxygen fueled; 9.8/10th full

---

[22] Eric Oetter on Joel Jamieson's website:

Most people stop at aerobic and anaerobic systems, but few break the anaerobic system down into the alactic and lactic branch. As The Myth of HIIT stresses, saying something "anaerobic" isn't nearly specific enough. Throwing a ball is predominantly anaerobic. Doing as many vertical jumps as possible in one minute is also predominantly anaerobic, but these activities are vastly different. Therefore, the logical conclusion to draw is that all anaerobic training is not created equally. 23

When you first begin intense activity, all three of the systems are activated. For the first 15-or-so seconds, the alactic anaerobic system is pumping hard, along with the others. But because it is only partially full, it runs out of gas fast.

Then the body promotes the Alactic Anaerobic system as the primary contributor given the movement intensity remains high. If you continue this activity, obviously there comes a time when the system will be depleted, at which point the aerobic bank supplies most of the energy. In this example, it is

[23] Mychal, Anthony. The Myth of HIIT. 22.

clear to see the aerobic system is the most efficient energy pathway.

With all of this lead in you are probably wondering, dreading even, what type of exercise I am going to prescribe because everyone knows running or walking on a treadmill for hours on end is not the most exciting thing in the world to do, even with a huge television screen in front of you. Right off the bat, I'll tell you right now that you will not be "training like a man" and "lifting heavy". No surprise there based on the last section, right? I'm still waiting for someone to explain how one can train like a man and look like a goddess if the men who train in the same manner don't.

When it comes to cardio, everyone claims to hate long steady state cardio and would rather HIIT for 10 - 15 minutes to satisfy their exercise requirement of the day. The problem with short HIIT workouts is that it can take up to twenty minutes for exercise to reduce insulin levels and lower blood sugar enough to enter, as in just starting, a fat burning zone. It has also been proven that after longer bouts of exercise (around the post 30-minute mark) endorphins start to get released and growth hormone (a fat burning furnace) and testosterone (muscle building) levels begin to rise. These levels continue to rise in a linear fashion over time, peaking around the 70-minute mark.

So, does this mean that in order to get your thigh gap and annihilate your body fat, you'll have to go down the marathon running path? Absolutely not! There is a big difference between aerobic training and marathon running. For the record, aerobic training also need not be either steady state or prolonged.

I should also state for the record, I have nothing against HIIT. All I care about is the appropriate manner of training that will burn the most fat and thus reveal the slim thighs you desire. Since many people tout HIIT as being the fat blasting cure-all, my job is to prove to you and set the record straight about the unadulterated facts.

Having said that, the fact is weight lifting cannot be our primary or sole means of exercising because it uses glucose/glycon and not fat when you engage in it. This does not mean that weight lifting isn't beneficial. We will use weight-bearing exercises, but since we want to target as much stored fat in our workout program, lifting isn't the most effective means to get us there. You are burning little to no fat during lifting and all glucose (glycogen) - the by product of using glycogen for energy in lactate acid which leads to swelling and soreness that peaks a day or two after the workout and resolves a few days later, depending on the severity of the damage.

Here's another fact: steady state cardio at a snail's pace and running like a madwoman every day isn't the solution either. Go ahead and heave a sigh of relief over that last line now.

In a 1993 study by Romajin and Colleagues, substrate metabolism was examined during different intensities of activity. The first one was 25% of VO2, the second was 65% of VO2, and the third, 85% of VO2. The result was very little difference between exercising at 25% VO2 and 85% VO2, meanwhile the 65% group showed the most mobilization of fat, or over triple the amounts as the other two groups.

In other words, the people that you spot gingerly walking on a treadmill while on the cell phone or reading all the articles in the latest gossip magazine and the people who are killing themselves burn roughly the same amount of fat, while those exercising in the middle range (not too slow, not too fast, but just right) burned three times as much fat! How can this be? This is because high intensity activity requires powerful muscle contractions of which carbohydrates are better at fueling than fats.

What about the fact that working out a higher intensity will burn more overall calories and the frequently heralded "after-effect" or Post-Exercise Oxygen Consumption (EPOC for short) of HIIT?

It is true that working out at a higher intensity will burn more total calories which will lead to faster fat loss, especially if you are eating low carbs and on a deficit. However, the small amount of total workout time for HIIT has been shown to equal the amount of calories burned doing lesser intensity workouts for a longer time. On top of that, you're prone to more injury and require lots of recovery time when you train very intensely, whereas spending a little more time working out at a moderate level can be done more often with less chance of injury.

As for those claims that HIIT will raise metabolism because the body will continually burn calories after the workout is over.

Are those calories being burned after the workout coming from fat? Sadly, the answer to that question is no. Those carbohydrates that are broken down inside the body are used for fuel after a HIIT session as well.

Furthermore, aerobic training also creates EPOC. But, EPOC for HIIT and Aerobic training is simply not a great calorie burner when one takes a closer look at things. With HIIT, you are getting a 14% EPOC, while with aerobic training, you are getting 7% EPOC. To put this into perspective, a 500-calorie burning working would have only a 35-calorie difference in EPOC. So much for getting that extra burn throughout the day.

HIIT is not all bad though; it may actually suppress your appetite, build more muscles than aerobic training, and muscles will raise your BMR as long as they are maintained.

THE THIGH GAP WORKOUT™

Okay, it may seem like we've covered a great deal of information, and we have because I want you to know the reasoning behind why you're going to do the protocol set forth below. I don't want to keep you waiting any longer, and you're probably itching for me to just spit out what you need to do already. Your wait is over, because you've reached the part of the book where you will finally learn the most effective workout combination and hacks to losing stubborn body fat without creating the swollen leg appearance.

My favorite analogy for fat loss is to see your body as a swimming pool, where the water is your body fat. You can't just take water out of the shallow end or the deep end. As you remove water initially, the overall level drops. Similarly, as you begin losing fat, you lose it everywhere. Eventually the only water left in the pool is in the deep end. In your body, the "deep end" for many women is usually the hips and thighs, as we know. You won't get rid of those until you've trimmed down everywhere else, for the most part (I'll explain this caveat in a minute).

Given that we have covered the various benefits of each type of training method, which type should we assume to reduce your overall body fat as quickly as possible, so that those stubborn areas can be targeted and finally start to slim down?

The answer is a training program that will build and maintain muscles where we want them, to keep your metabolism raised, burn the most fat while taking into account your lowered carbohydrate diet, not result in an increase in mass or muscular look in the thigh region (hypertrophy and sarcoplasmic fluid), and burn as many calories as possible without negatively affecting your appetite.

A combination of exercises tailored around your calorie cycling days will yield all of the above. Cardio alone won't burn as many calories as higher intensity interval training. It also won't maintain existing muscles that will keep your metabolism raised without any extra effort on your part. It will however, burn a greater percentage of fat and can be done more frequently (at a moderate pace) without fear of injury.

On the other hand, higher intensity training the way you're meant to do it (for 15 to 20 minutes) will limit the frequency you are able to work out due to the recovery period necessary, burn as much calories as moderate intensity training done for a little bit longer and most people don't train at the true intensity levels required. Still, it will build more muscle and keep your metabolism up.

THIGH GAP PROTOCOL TO LOSE FAT

Remember all the way back in the first few chapters when we discussed different solutions for your unique problem? We're going to pick back up where we left off and begin with what you'll need to do if fat loss is your primary concern. Note that while you may elect to develop your own workout program, since I will provide you with the "how to" below, by becoming a member of "The Thigh Gap Club" you can have access to new, full 'Thigh Gap Workouts" every month, with everything already planned out for you. Variety and switching up your exercises is integral to preventing fat loss plateau and combating boredom. Visit www.thighgaphack.com/products or www.thighgapclub.com for more information.

In this protocol, you will be required to train a minimum of four and a maximum of six days per week, depending on your current fitness level, alternating workout intensity. The number of training days will depend on your current fitness level, with beginners starting at four days per week, and more advanced individuals jumping right in with six workout days per week. If training four days, you will cycle two days on, one day off, two days on, two days off and so on. If training five days, you will cycle two days on, and one day off. Six days will translate to three days on, one day off and so on. I will explain the why behind this type of training in the exercise cycling section below.

The following example illustrates how one would approach workouts and intensity levels on a six day schedule: Mon – higher intensity workout, Tues – Moderate intensity workout, Wed – Higher intensity workout, Thurs – Rest, Fri – Moderate intensity workout, Sat – Higher intensity Workout, Sunday – Moderate intensity workout. By steering clear of killer intensity workouts like Tabata and Crossfit, you can workout more regularly and take less time recovering, which translates to more calories burned.

Your workouts will utilize interval circuit training using full body compound movements to burn as many calories as possible. You will incorporate compound resistance training movements of the upper and lower body for thirty to forty five minutes to preserve existing lean mass, which will keep your BMR elevated, and end your workout sessions with moderate to high intensity cardio for another thirty to forty five minutes. Doing cardio right after your training will keep nutrients needed for growth out of your system in your most anabolic window. On your lighter intensity workout days, you can choose to forego resistance/circuit training altogether and just complete cardio for the entire sixty-minute workout or do a modified version of your higher by doing less sets, reps or going at a slower pace.

Begin by picking out exercises that involve compound movements with different intensities. Compound movements use more than one muscle at a time to burn more calories. An example would be completing overhead presses with alternating front kicks instead of just doing an overhead press by itself, which would be an isolation movement. Again, for a tailored plan that includes specific exercises, look into joining our online community.

You will need to switch from one exercise to the next without resting (circuit training) while varying the intensity enough to catch your breath and keep going (interval training). Leg exercises can be a combination of bigger fat burning movements and smaller muscle targeting exercises.

The large lower body fat burning exercises would be plies, front, side and back kicks, backward/side/curtsy lunges, wide squats and deadlifts with body weight or three to five pound weights. These should be higher reps and done no more than three times per week with two rest days in between. Small pulsing leg movements typically work the tiny muscles in the hips, thighs and butt from different angles by lifting, extending or bending the leg or knee. You may do these with high reps (50 to 100 per set) with no to low weights to train the muscle fibers responsible for endurance, which do not increase in size. Leg pulsing exercises where you work the smaller muscles can be done up to six days per week for twenty to thirty minutes, and can be engage the upper body (arms lifted, arm circles, arm pulses, etc).

You should try to avoid exercises that require lying down completely, as more energy is expended when you are upright or your body is contracted. It is important for these exercises to get your heart rate up because that is how you burn calories, so if you're barely breaking a sweat, exert more effort and up the intensity.

Cardio, which is to be completed at the end of each workout, can either be done using a cardio dvd or exercise plan, like the ones updated regularly in "The Thigh Gap Workout", or walking on a treadmill, without holding on, at a moderate but non-panting pace and a moderate incline. You can gauge whether you are doing your walk correctly if you are sweating buckets and feel your abs slightly engaged. Long strides that will stretch the legs are best. I particularly like dance cardio and kickboxing for my cardio, but feel free to switch up your routines as you see fit.

All of the above should be done in conjunction with a warm up/cool down period with ample stretching of the limbs every day, as well as a low carb, calorie deficit diet outlined in the diet and food hacks section to really maximize fat burning and prevent hypertrophy of the muscles. You can lessen the deficit or elect to eat at maintenance on workout days and increase the deficit on rest days, but doing so will lead to slower fat loss albeit give you more energy to put into your workouts.

THIGH GAP PROTOCOL TO LOSE MUSCLE

For the lot of you with athletic builds facing overdeveloped muscles, chances are high a contributing factor to your bulky muscles is underlying fat. This is not to dismiss some women's ability to develop muscles very easily. You very well could have a preponderance of muscle, but we must acknowledge fat being a highly likely contributor to your circumstance.

Therefore, before we go into this protocol, be sure that you are already lean and the muscles in your legs are not just excess fat, as maintaining your muscles when you have excess fat to lose will keep your metabolism higher and allow you to burn more fat. In other words, if you get rid of muscles and you have a lot of fat to lose, you'll be putting yourself at a grave disadvantage.

Like The Thigh Gap Protocol for fat loss, your version of the Protocol requires a sizeable calorie deficit, stretching every day, and upper body resistance training four to six times per week for thirty to forty five minutes to maintain lean body mass. However, you will need to complete a non-negotiable cardio regimen of 6 days per week in a fasted state and work the accessory muscles in the legs using endurance training (high rep/no weight) stopping short of failure, after cardio. You may choose to split up your upper body training and fasted cardio work at different times in the day.

Also, whereas those who have a lot of fat to lose or who do not put on muscle as easily can incorporate some of the more traditional calorie burning exercises such as backward, curtsy and side lunges, deadlifts, and squats two to three times a week, your regimen will require complete omission of leg resistance training, as doing any of the aforementioned moves (even without weights) will serve to maintain the lean muscle in your lower body that you want to diminish.

You will complete low to moderate impact cardio every day for thirty to forty five minutes at the start (4 – 6 weeks) and progress to sixty minutes towards the end of the program (6 – 12 weeks). The reason for extending your sessions is your body adapts to steady state cardio over time by burning less calories. Some cardio that require explosive movements, like interval sprinting and plyometric exercises, will have the exact opposite effect on your muscles, so stick to walking on a treadmill with no to low incline at a non-panting pace or other forms of low impact cardio.

Immediately follow cardio training with twenty to thirty or so minutes of endurance training movements that work the slow twitch muscle fibers in the lower body (think along the lines of small pulsing movements instead of full range leg exercises or join our membership community for access to full routine videos). Aim for two sets of 50 reps, where you complete one set of each exercise on one leg before switching to the next leg, and then repeating it all over again. Keep in mind, 'toning' exercises such as this only works when there is little body fat as blood flow influences fat storage and loss.

Finally, and this is key, you are not to consume protein (that includes shakes) for three to four hours after working out, as protein replenishes and rebuilds your muscle. A cup of green tea or salad (without any meat) after your workout is best.

Working your legs in this manner will not only burn fat and break down excess muscles, but also prevent mass from occurring. If you're concerned that walking will make your legs bigger, don't be. Resistance training causes hypertrophy, not walking. You also don't want to stop all lower body work altogether, as some may advocate, or the result will be fat, squishy looking legs instead of lean ones. When you stop using the muscles in your legs in the manner your body has become accustomed to, eventually it will realize it has no need for the muscles and use it up.

A final word of caution on the Thigh Gap Protocol for muscle loss is you have to really eat clean and avoid high carb and high sugar snacks because less muscle will lead to a slower metabolism that may encourage fat storage in unwanted places. You should also follow this diet and training regimen for no more than eight to twelve weeks, after which you may cut down on exercise time/frequency, but do not return to high resistance leg exercises (squats, lunges, explosive leg movements, etc) which caused you to put on a ton of muscles in the legs in the first place.

WORKOUT CYCLING

One of the secrets to my thigh gap workout hack is timing and it is to be applied whether you need to lose fat or muscle. You are to rotate your workouts to take advantage of prime fat burning opportunities. Thus, I recommend working out back to back days in the following pattern: at night one day, and in the morning (fasted) the immediate day. For example, if you were a beginner working out 4 times per week, your schedule would be as follows: Monday night three to four hours after your last meal, Tuesday morning fasted, rest Wednesday, Thursday night three to four hours after your last meal, Friday morning fasted, rest Saturday and Sunday. It is completely fine to do your lower intensity training on fasted morning workout days for the Thigh Gap Protocol for Fat Loss.

Why do I advocate training in this manner? There are those that say you burn more fat when you work out after a fast and others that say working out right after a meal works best so that your body will have to use the calories you consume to fuel that workout instead of storing it as fat.

What is important to know is that your body is in either a "fed" or "fasted" state. When your body is in a fed state it primarily uses carb-energy for fuel, unless you are fat adapted. When your body is in a fasted state it releases HGH. This hormone helps release body fat from stored fat cells into the bloodstream so you can use that for energy instead of stored "food energy". Intense exercise also raises HGH levels. When you combine exercise with this fasted state, you create a great synergistic condition for fat loss. Obviously you can't overdo this and fast for way too long or exercise too hard, but done strategically this works wonders.

To summarize, whether you work out morning, noon or night, try to do so when your body is in a fasted state. The longer the fasted state, the better, but waiting 3 or 4 hours after eating before working out will do the trick.

HACK TIPS

GREEN TEA AND EXERCISE

How did Green Tea get into the exercise portion of the book? Simple. Consuming green tea before and after a workout instead of a carb or protein filled shake will increase fat loss like crazy!

WORKOUT RIGHT BEFORE EATING

Recall our discussion, if you will, on energy (Calories) you take going to your muscles and once they are full being stored as fat cells. One hack, which I credit Tim Ferriss for sharing, is effective at circumventing body fat from being stored in the first place.

According to Ferriss, working out merely minutes before eating a meal is the answer. Surprisingly, the workout does not have to be 30 minutes, 20 minutes or even 10 minutes long.

Five minutes of rigorous exercise is all it takes to sufficiently deplete the muscles of energy. The exercise Ferriss recommends is wall squats. However, exhausting these muscles and then supply your body energy to repair the leg muscles is not exactly aligned to getting slender pins. Instead, I recommend doing a few sets of pushups or upper/lower back exercises for five minutes with light weights.

SWEAT TO SLIM

Back in the day I would go to the park to work out and see people wearing what appeared to be a garbage bag sweat suits or tons of heavy, hot looking clothes while working out. I didn't understand what those 'kooky' people were trying to do then, but now I know they were trying to eliminate water weight. Just as those who embark on a low carb diet see rapid weight loss in the first few weeks due to loss of water weight, working out in those garbage bag sweat suits and heavy clothing can accomplish the same end thing.

For this to work most effectively, you need to open the pores before working out with sauna suit. A cream that works extremely well is called Albolene, it's a moisturizing cleanser but it really opens your pores up and allows you to sweat more freely. Some also have reported applying menthol to the skin before suiting up and working out.

Today, there are more fashionable and less 'kooky', attention drawing, options for someone looking to get the benefits of sweating to slim. You can pick up a suit at a sporting goods store for around $20. Alternatively, you could purchase clothing online. Again, refer to the resources page for a list of vendors I recommend. (www.thighgaphack.com/resources)

WEIGHTED CLOTHING

One thing you should keep in mind as you attempt to contour your body is, the more weight you lose the lower your metabolism will be due to your body not requiring as much energy and effort to be moved. As a rule of thumb, the more muscles you have or heavier you are, the higher your BMR or the Calories you burn when at rest. The bigger your calorie deficit and the more weight or muscles you lose, the lower your BMR will be.

One suggestion for combating your lowered metabolism as you star to lose weight is to work out in weighted clothing. Imagine walking up a hill with 10 pounds weights vs. no weights. One would take considerably more amounts of energy and exertion. Wearing a weighted vest (about 10 percent of your body weight) while walking can boost your calorie burn by 8 percent.

Too many weighted vests look bulky and unfashionable, but I have found a few companies that have taken fashion and appearance into mind in their designs. Let's face it, if you feel like a fool wearing the weighted vests/clothes you are less likely to actually ever use them. For a list of companies I recommend, visit www.thighgaphack.com/resources

EXERCISES TO AVOID

These various exercise hacks were sourced from a few smart and well-respected personal trainers and it relates particularly well for our purposes of slimming down your thighs by avoiding certain exercises and replacing them with other more effective ones.

An exercise that women are often told to do when trying to lose fat or muscles is forward lunges, in which you extend one leg at a ninety degree angle, while stretching the other leg as straight as possible before returning to a standing position.

Forward lunges actually build up the base at the front part of the kneecap, specifically the vastus medialus creating what is commonly called the overhang or teardrop effect. While the teardrop looks great on men, most women I know would rather this muscle remain in hiding. In that same vein, doing a leg press, where you incline on a machine and push weight up with both feet, especially with heavy weights, will work the same area and give you that very developed muscle that you do not want.

Instead, I prescribe replacing forward lunges and leg extensions with backward lunges, where you step back with one leg and bring the knee to a 90-degree angle. The angles of your backward lunges matter because of the muscles that are engaged when you go further into the lunge. When you do backward lunges, your butt gets a lot more work, and the section of the quads that run up and down the length of the femur (rectus femoris) get a bit more work.

This doesn't mean you can never do a forward lunge again (although I would recommend staying away from the leg press and opting for using body weight when it comes to legs) but you should cut down on them significantly and where they are called for in workout videos simply opt for the backward lunge. When you do decide to incorporate front lunges make sure to only use body weight as additional weights exacerbate the problem. The same applies for backward lunges.

In the same vein, traditional low squats also should be avoided because they will increase the quadriceps and hips. Wider squat stances are preferable because they increase glute recruitment and take the quads out just a bit more than regular front squats. Jump lunges are okay since you catch evenly with both legs lessening the effect and step ups are also okay, because people tend to use the training leg. By driving through the HEEL of the elevated foot when completing step ups, you force more recruitment of the glute and hamstrings than the quad.

Part 7 - Outside Hacks

DIGGING DEEPER

You may be wondering what a chapter that doesn't have to deal with diet or exercise is doing in this book. I am a total advocate and living proof of what smart dieting and exercise can help you achieve in contouring your total body. However, this book is called 'The Thigh Gap Hack" with the sub-title "Learn Every Trick in the Book, literally - for thinner thighs and slim, toned legs". I promised to tell you all the secrets to accomplish your thigh gap goal, so my work is not yet done.

My job is to give you every tool I have found that works and for you to decide which ones to use and trash the rest. Thus, I have compiled some of the little known secrets and tricks that many celebrities and fitness athletes have used throughout the years to slim down their thighs, some being quick temporary fixes and others long term, simply because they work.

LEG WRAPS

Leg Wraps, a specific form of Body wraps, permit you to shed inches via water reduction (water is a pound per pint) and are short-term solutions to lose inches. When you might wish to look your very best but there is hardly any time for you to reduce weight, they can be very effective.

Having a leg wrap isn't as risky as having a full-body wrap, which can cause overheating and excessive fluid loss that may lead to dehydration. A leg wrap to decrease the size of your thighs involves wrapping your legs and thighs in compression bandages, which may be nothing more than ace bandages infused with oils, herbs and minerals. Many DIY solutions call for regular plastic wrap, foil, vinyl, seaweed, clay, or mud.

Depending on where you have your leg wrap done, you can expect to spend an hour or so relaxing, or you may be required to get in a little time on the treadmill while your thighs are heating up and shrinking. Coupling leg wraps with the hacks provided in this book (proper eating and exercise) can produce fabulous results. For a list of recommended reputable wrap companies and promotions, visit the Thigh Gap Resources Page at www.thighgaphack.com/resources

MASSAGES

There are two types of massages that can assist in weight loss, but not fat loss, there is a difference. The first type of massage is called a lymphatic massage that takes the focus off your muscles. The lymphatic system is a complex network of fluid-filled tubes that continuously bathe our cells and then carries away the body's "sewage" (toxins, waste liquid) to filters called lymph nodes, where harmful substances are trapped and neutralized. Lymph nodes are all over your body.

We are said to have three times more lymph fluid than blood in the body, but while blood has the heart to pump and keep blood moving, lymphs rely on the movement of muscles to provide a pump for lymphatic fluid. Other factors, such as stress, illness, pollution, pesticides in food and chemicals overload and stall the lymph system, which leads to fluid back up and bloating.

Lymphatic drainage is a light massage that uses gentle, rhythmic strokes to free up the fluids in your lymph nodes, allowing it to leave the body, and thus releasing weight in the form of dead cells and fluids. If you can't afford yourself a series of lymphatic drainage massage treatments, do them by yourself! Use your favorite cream and massage it twice a day onto your legs with small upward circular movements to stimulate circulation.

Besides water weight loss and reduced bloating and swelling, some added benefits of releasing lymphs to flow freely are more nutrients are able to get to the cells, more calories become energy, clearer and smooth skin, and lessened cravings. The long, smooth friction associated with lymphatic drainage massage can also break up the adipose pockets, bound tissue and sub-cutaneous scar tissue that create cellulite. Other DIY tips for getting the lymph fluid moving is to dry brush the skin and/or jump on a mini trampoline, also known as rebounding.

Secondly, regular massages (especially deep massage) have quite an impact on various systems of the body. Depending on the nature of the massage and the skills & knowledge of the therapist, it will amongst other things stimulate blood circulation and lymph flow, and improve breathing and digestion - and improvements here will have a beneficial impact on other functions. In effect it is like performance tuning - the body will generally start operating more efficiently.

LIPO ALTERNATIVES

Liposuction alternative will not produce results as drastic as liposuction and are not intended for people who are obese. These body-contouring procedures are for fit individuals with stubborn areas of fat. Namely, the following procedures can be helpful in targeting thigh fat if you don't feel comfortable working to lower your body fat further through diet and exercise:

Exposure to Cold – Cryolipolysis, popularly known as CoolSculpting (ZELTIQ), refers to a medical device used to destroy fat cells. A typical CoolSculpting session lasts 60 minutes and costs approximately $700 (doctors are charged by the manufacturer approximately $110 per session). During the procedure the doctor gently pinches the fatty area between the

CoolSculpting applicator arms to extract energy (cooling) from the underlying fat tissue without damage to other tissues. The applicator cup uses a gentle vacuum pressure to draw the tissue between the cooling panels.

We've discussed cold therapy before, and this is precisely what this procedure uses for results. When fat cells are exposed to precise cooling, they trigger a process of natural removal that gradually reduces the thickness of the fat layer.

Light Waves – Low-level laser therapy is defined as treatment with a dose rate that causes no immediate detectable temperature rise of the treated tissues and no macroscopically visible changes in tissue structure. The most popular form of this therapy is Zerona, which works by aiming lasers at your lower body specifically designed to puncture holes in your fat cells so that they deflate. Your body keeps all the fat cells, but they are said to be much smaller.

Radio Waves (radiofrequency) – Velashape is one of the more popular procedures that uses radiofrequency. From the company's website: "Vacuum and specially designed rollers for the Mechanical Massage smooth out the skin to facilitate safe and efficient heat energy delivery. The net result increases the metabolism of stored energy, increases lymphatic drainage and reduces or shrinks the size of the actual fat cells and fat chambers."

Sound Waves (ultrasound) – Liposonix is one of several treatments approved by the FDA that uses ultrasound technology to melt fat. Eventually, a slow death of the fat cells occur (the cell themselves are absorbed and do not return). The procedure can last up to an hour and a half and costs between $1,500 and $3,000 per session. Full results can take 6-to-12 weeks.

A relatively newer procedure that involved ultrasound is called "Ultrasound Cavitation". The ultrasound wavelength quickly expands and contracts (vibrates) the cell membrane of the fat cell causing a small air pocket to develop inside the cell. This air bubble then bursts the cell wall and the triglycerides inside the cell are released into the surrounding fluid (interstitial fluid). The cost is about $350 per session. When having this procedure done you will hear a sound, so keep that in mind to make sure you're not being taken for a ride.

Regardless of which procedure you decide upon, remember that they are no single (or combination) of treatment will be a miracle cures and should be used as complimentary medicine, not a cure all. I would also recommend working out, particularly with long low to moderate intensity walking sessions, directly after having any alternative lipo treatment to help rid your body of the fat released and floating around in the body. Of course, consult with your doctor beforehand to make sure that working out after treatment is safe.

HERBS

Yohimbe (yohimbine HCL) is a herb that helps with fat mobilization in stubborn body fat areas such as women' hips and thighs. However, it is not effective for those who are not already relatively lean. It is best to take yohimbe right before doing aerobic exercise.

Then there is ephedrine. Known as the EC stack,. Some of you may be alarmed because the herbal form of ephedra was banned in due to the misuse of the substance. Normally combined with combine dieters ignored the guidelines for how much and how frequent to take EC stacks and thus suffered consequences, which included death. I hesitate to even include this but ephedrine is effective.

However, and this is where I want you to really listen to me so that you don't end up being one of the unfortunate who disregard instructions and pay the price, EC and yohimbe should NEVER be mixed together. It is recommended that you do not take EC or Yohimbe within hours of each other, because otherwise the side effects of each can cause serious elevated heart rate and blood pressure.

STRETCHING

Muscle does one of two things, contracts or elongates. Muscles that are contracted under load become resistant to elongation by involuntarily remaining partially contracted. The more you contract your muscles the less willing they are to elongate fully, especially in the complex joints of the hips and shoulders. Often the more your try to elongate the muscle the stronger the involuntary contraction becomes making it impossible to elongate the muscle fully. Certain exercises, like Yoga and Pilates, apply gentle force to the muscles to overcome these involuntary contractions thus allowing the muscle to more fully elongate. Deep and long stretching also allows you to fully elongate your muscles.

The idea behind Yoga and Pilates is you can lengthen and elongate the muscle through deep muscle strengthening, while relaxing and not overworking the "big" surface muscles. The imagery of length combined with better posture helps to produce the desired overall effect as well. This is why I recommend steering clear or greatly reducing exercises that work the big leg muscles such as squats and lunges in both Thigh Gap Protocols.

While, you can't actually change the length of your muscles, it's hard to refute obvious results Yoga and Pilates practitioners boast when they combine their form of exercise with a sensible diet. To mimic their results, stretch immediately after working out (no exceptions), and try to get into the habit of stretching upon waking up and right before going to sleep for fifteen or so minutes each time. Search for leg stretches on the Internet and try to hold each stretch for at least 30 seconds.

FOAM ROLLING

Along the same lines of a massage is foam rolling. Foam Rolling has becoming very popular as of late. Foam rollers not only stretches muscles and tendons but it also breaks down soft tissue adhesions and scar tissue. By using your own body weight and a cylindrical foam roller you can perform a self-massage or myofascial release, break up trigger points, and soothe tight fascia while increasing blood flow and circulation to the soft tissues.

When you roll onto a spot of discomfort, the idea is to pause on that spot for 30-60 seconds each for the desired inhibition to take effect. After a workout, foam rolling can: relax shortened muscle tissue, increase circulation to the tissue and increase venous and lymphatic drainage,

Part 8 – Motivation Hacks

HOW TO REMAIN MOTIVATED

STOP RIGHT THERE! Don't be tempted to skip over this section thinking you have everything you need. The majority of people's fitness incentives fail not because they don't want results, but because it is difficult to consistently do anything that requires work and discipline.

Everyone has days when they don't feel like working out, or someone brings cookies into the office and you don't feel like being the only one having to restrain yourself. One would think, if gains (or losses) are being made, it would be motivation enough to keep up whatever is causing the success. However, the phenomenon of people losing sight of their goals and not seeing their programs through doesn't only occur when results are slow or hard to see.

Sometimes even though a person could be seeing obvious results, they become complacent and start to slack off.

Therefore, I have included what I call "motivation hacks" you can refer to whenever you realize you are beginning to feel unmotivated to work out or eat properly. These tricks will get your intention back to where it needs to be.

BE HELD ACCOUNTABLE

Become the leader of some sort of fitness group like Zumba, BeachBody or even a meetup group. It's hard not to show up to work out when you're the leader and people are depending on you. You are also more likely to give it everything you've got when you're trying to motivate other people. As an instructor, even on weeks when you really don't want to exercise, you at least have to show up for the few classes you teach. Many can attest to just showing up being the hardest part; once you're there and start going through the motions, you'd be amazed at how quickly the energy of others will cause your lackluster attitude and energy to kick in.

Alternatively, you could sign up for one or multiple marathons and races, like Tough Mudder or race walking events. If you are concerned about running, which I don't particularly enjoy, sign up for a bikini or fitness competition, beauty pageant, or any of the number of fitness contests online that boast very attractive prizes. Our very own "Feminine Contour Fitness Competition", and list of prizes, can be found at www.thefemininecontour.com/competition and our 'Thigh Gap Hack Competition' along with prizes, can be found at www.thighgaphack.com/competition

We also keep an updated list of fitness competitions from all across the web at www.thighgaphack.com/resources

While training for a thigh gap can be enough for some people, others would do well to introduce a competitive element to keep them motivated. Also, once you commit money of your own or raise money, especially if it's for a cause you believe in, you'll have an added incentive to stick to your training regimen. This strategy is even more effective if you've got friends willing to commit and train for the race or event with you.

FIGHT BOREDOM

If you are a fan of workout DVD's, like I am, you may be a familiar with a little something called exercise boredom. Whether you simply get bored with having to listen to the same dialogue, music or watch the same scenery over and over again, or have felt the ire of having to sit through portions of workouts that you aren't too fond of to get to the good part, you can start to dread and thus lose all motivation to complete your workouts.

A means of overcoming such instances is to use any blank DVD or external hard drive and Hardbrake to break the DRM, and then use Windows Live MovieMaker or any other editing software to remix the workout routines into a 30-minute program tailored to your needs. I prefer using an external hard drive for all of my workout videos as it makes organizing and access to working out excruciatingly easy.

You can also do something similar with Youtube.com workout videos by creating an account and making a custom workout playlist or searching for other people's workout playlist. One trick when using YouTube is to custom your search by hitting the search tools function bar and selecting videos greater than 20 minutes and/or newly uploaded videos. We've taken the liberty of putting together a huge list of the best YouTube workout channels on the youtube page www.youtube.com/thighgaphack as well as on our resources page www.thefemininecontour.com/resources

Finally, there are communities you can join for free or a small fee, where you can access new workout videos every week. Our very own community, "The Feminine Contour", is highly recommended. We post new full-segment length cardio dance, toning, resistance training and general fitness related videos every week. Joining our community is completely free and as simple as signing up at www.thefemininecontour.com

AUDIO BOOKS

This may be quite a common one, but when exercising outdoors on a repetitive route or on a piece of exercise equipment, fight boredom by listening to audio books with topics that you find intriguing. The content of the books should interest you enough for the time to seemingly fly by.

LOGGED IN

Set your password for your work computer, email, facebook, twitter and any other logins that you type every day or multiples times a day to something motivational that will remind you of a goal. Some simple examples you can use are "Th*gh G@p", "th!n th!gh$", "e@t L3ss", and "@lmost rac3 day".

EAT WITH YOUR NON-DOMINANT HAND

Start trying to use your non-dominant hand during various daily activities such as eating and brushing your teeth. Forcing yourself out of normal habitual patterns activates certain parts of the brain, which may contribute to improving willpower.

GO TO BED IN FITNESS GEAR

Particularly useful for those early morning fasted state workouts, is this hack of going to bed in workout clothes and ensuring other apparel/accessories you'll need (sports bra, socks, sneakers) are close by or at the door. If you use an alarm on your phone to wake you up, put it on top of your duffel bag or workout DVD. If you use a computer, pre-load the video on your laptop screen, so it's the first thing you see and only requires you to press play to begin.

Waking up knowing that you not only need to work out, but also need to sleepily pack a bag or figure out which workout to do can be disheartening. It can be tough to get up and get dressed when it's super early, still dark out, and your partner is still cozy in bed, trying to sleep. Readying yourself for your morning workout not only keeps you from rummaging around in the morning, potentially disturbing your partner, and minimizes the amount of time needed to get dressed, which equates to more sleep, it also motivates and guilt-trips you into actually working out.

The unavoidable guilt from waking up in or near your fitness gear, and having to take it off after failing to actually utilize it, works surprisingly well to hold people accountable.

SOMETHING TO LOOK FORWARD TO

All too common, the only time women tend to be exceedingly motivated to get in shape is for a very important upcoming event, such as a wedding, high school or family reunion, vacation, party, etc. They crash diet for a few weeks and then once the event is over, they slack off and go back to their old habits.

By having a very social and active lifestyle, which requires attendance at special events and/or functions where you want to stun in a particular outfit, you will have a great excuse to constantly be on top of your diet and fitness game.

Just because you are currently lacking invitations to such functions, doesn't mean you can't easily seek them out, especially if you live in a large city. It is completely possible to orchestrate a full social calendar by joining organizations and club, and/or arranging galas, parties, charity functions, etc. You could also be the host and throw a party or gathering. Don't think you have to find something to do every week or weekend, aim for one to two special functions a month to give you something worth looking great to.

THINSPIRATION

Yes, looking at beautiful pictures of slender women can be motivating to some, but to others such pictures are just a constant reminder of how far away they are from their goal. If thinspiration websites and pictures that feature beautiful women keep you on your diet and exercise program, then by all means utilize it. However, if thinspiration has the opposite effect on you, maybe it's time to try some negative reinforcement.

Nothing prevents me from eating something I know I shouldn't be eating than seeing someone currently dealing with the consequences of eating that very thing. I'm not saying you should go seeking out those pictures of overweight men and women with disparaging messages on them, but pictures embodying exactly what you don't want to become, or if you've made progress, go back to, can help thwart moments of weakness and help you resist temptations.

Another alternative to explore that may be effective is different, yet similar to conventional thinspiration, but more personalized. www.weightmirror.com is an online application that lets you upload your own photos and see yourself thinner. You can upload a picture and instantly view what you would look 10 to 50 pounds lighter. The app is currently free, but if you've got some Photoshop skills, you can make your own creations by cropping that can serve as fodder for diet and exercise motivation.

POSITIVE FITNESS AFFIRMATIONS

Finally, when you feel your motivation start to suffer from a slump, try positive affirmations to get you back on track. Since the average person has about sixty thousand thoughts per day, and 80 percent of those thoughts are negative, it's easy to see how we can be our biggest saboteurs.

Stating positive facts aloud to yourself has a powerful effect on your sub-conscious. Talking about the muscles that you are going to work and imagining the effect of the exercise on the muscle helps to give you the ultimate workout advantage. Your mind focuses on that particular muscle and triggers the appropriate hormonal release to allow you the most benefit.

To use the power of affirmations in your workouts, write down as many positive statements as you can about what you intend to do and eat and the wonderful effects you feel from completing these tasks. Examples of positive affirmations are:

I love making time to exercise and the way exercise makes me feel

My body is responding to my fitness goals

My spirit soars after I exercise

I am amazed at my own abilities

I will walk/workout for 15 additional minutes today

I am looking and feeling better every day

Read them aloud whenever you are feeling unmotivated, as well as speak positive words during your workout (e.g. – "I can feel the fat melting from my inner thighs"). Visualize your fat taking a beating, liquefying and being vaporized into thin air as you do your cardio routine. In your minds eye envision your legs slimming and thinning with each long stride you take. Try this simple, but very effective hack, and watch how your attitude can influence your stick-to-itiveness when it comes to employing the tactics in this book.

OUTSOURCE YOUR FITNESS

I can see your ears perking up now as you wonder how in the world I'm going to pull of a recommendation to outsource fitness. You and I both know you can't actually get someone to do your workouts for you, but the idea of outsourcing doesn't have to only be limited to business related work.

Outsourcing stands to make your life easier whether it be in the form of hiring a personal trainer to motivate you, signing up for food delivery programs or grocery lists tailored to specific healthy meals for the week. I'd say most clients hire personal trainers, not to help them exercise but as motivation to simply come into the gym. Commitment to another is often stronger than commitment to one's self, and even more so when money is involved.

Knowing this, I do urge anyone interested to reach out and contact me if they would like personalized services, whether it be meal planning, shopping lists, or custom workout plans. Feel free to e-mail me directly at Camille@thighgaphack.com with your inquiries and questions or sign up for any such program at http://www.thefemininecontour.com/products

I welcome your thoughts on the book and would love to receive pictures of your transformation as well!

###

WHERE DO YOU GO FROM HERE?

If you enjoyed this book, it would mean the world to me if you would please take a moment to write an honest review on Amazon.com, because that will help others know what they're going to get, check this book out, and get the same benefits you've achieved. I strongly believe that this information will help change people's lives, and you can help too by spreading the word.

Please also feel free to write a review on my (and your) facebook and twitter pages. While you're at it, like The Thigh Gap Hack on facebook, pinterest, tumblr, instagram and/or twitter and spread the word by sharing the content (workouts, articles, etc.) on your social network – including your own blogs and other healthy/diet/fitness/wellness blogs that you frequent!

If you felt this book could be better in any way, you can also let me know what could use improvement by sending an email to info@thighgaphack.com or camille@thighgaphack.com so I can update this and future books to best meet your needs and ensure everyone reading this will get the most value possible.

Looking for more health and fitness tips?

Besides the resources I have provided in this book, you'll want to check out my blog, youtube channel and newsletter with more tips and tricks at:

The Feminine Contour

www.thefemininecontour.com

www.youtube.com/thefemininecontour.com

www.twitter.com/thefemininecontour

www.facebook.com/thefemininecontour

THE THIGH GAP HACK

www.thighgaphack.com

http://www.thighgaphack.com

www.youtube.com/thighgaphack.com

www.facebook.com/thighgaphack.com

www.twitter.com/thighgaphack

Looking for a specific exercise and diet program for fat loss, health and/or muscle gain? Then make sure you order my brand new workout dvd, 'Bye-Bye Thunder Thighs', (to be released mid-march 2014).

It's a one hour long workout that combines stretching, toning and cardio exercises to melt the fat from your body and sculpt feminine, sexy thighs. You'll love the results you'll get – I promise! Go to http://www.thighgaphack.com/byebyethunderthighs to learn more

There's a lot of hype and gimmicky products out there when it comes to diets and exercise programs promising to get people to burn fat and get a "thigh gap" or "slimmer thighs". That being said, there are a few courses I highly recommend. The list is always being updated at www.thighgaphack.com/resources and at my blogs

www.thighgaphack.com

www.thighgaphack.com/blog   and
www.thefemininecontour.com/blog

21418921R00142

Made in the USA
San Bernardino, CA
19 May 2015